DESIGNER
NAILS

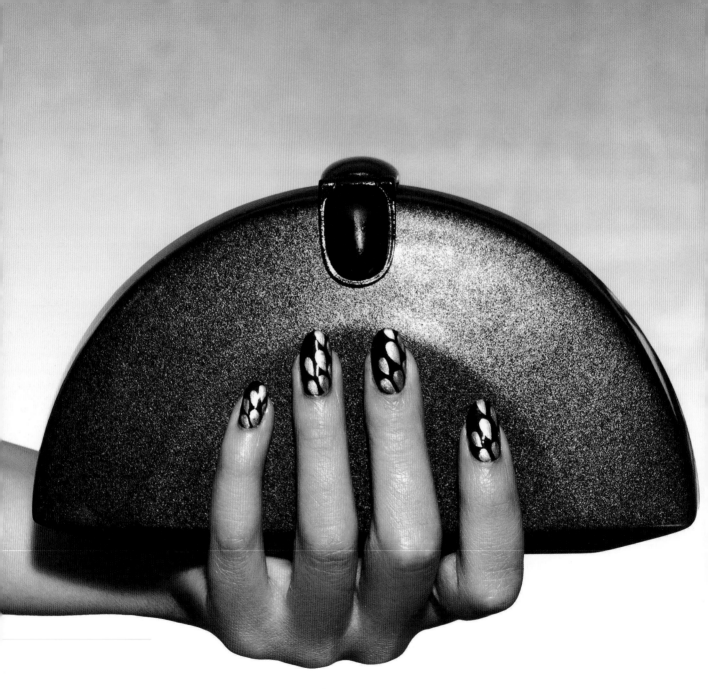

DESIGNER NAILS

CREATE ART AT YOUR FINGERTIPS

AMI VEGA

with Marisa Bulzone

A Perigee Book

PERIGEE

An imprint of Penguin Random House LLC

375 Hudson Street, New York, New York 10014

DESIGNER NAILS

ISBN: 978-0-399-17364-6

Page xi and 134: nail polishes © combomambo/iStock
Pages xvii, 133, and 137: nail polish spills © Foonia/iStock

This book has been registered with the Library of Congress.

First edition: August 2015

PRINTED IN THE UNITED STATES OF AMERICA

10 9 8 7 6 5 4 3 2 1

Text design by Georgia Rucker
Photographs by Jason Setiawan

Neither the publisher nor the author is engaged in rendering professional advice or services to
the individual reader. The ideas, procedures, and suggestions contained in this book are not intended
as a substitute for consulting with your physician. All matters regarding your health require medical
supervision. Neither the author nor the publisher shall be liable or responsible for any loss or damage
allegedly arising from any information or suggestion in this book.

While the author has made every effort to provide accurate telephone numbers, Internet
addresses, and other contact information at the time of publication, neither the publisher nor the
author assumes any responsibility for errors, or for changes that occur after publication. Further,
the publisher does not have any control over and does not assume any responsibility for author
or third-party websites or their content.

Most Perigee books are available at special quantity discounts for bulk purchases for sales
promotions, premiums, fund-raising, or educational use. Special books, or book excerpts, can also
be created to fit specific needs. For details, write: SpecialMarkets@penguinrandomhouse.com.

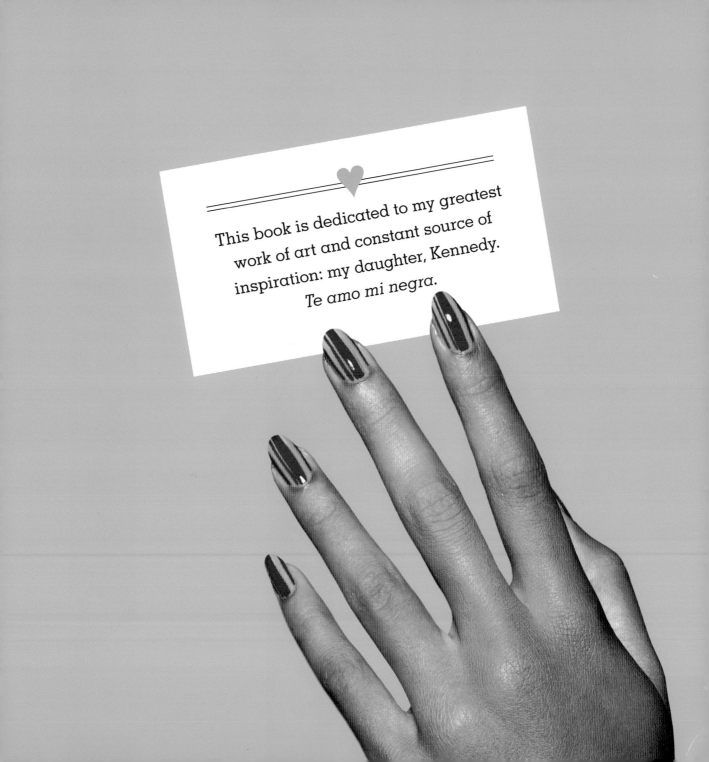

This book is dedicated to my greatest work of art and constant source of inspiration: my daughter, Kennedy.

Te amo mi negra.

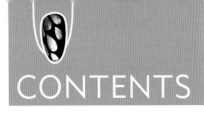

CONTENTS

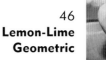

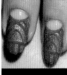

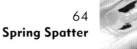

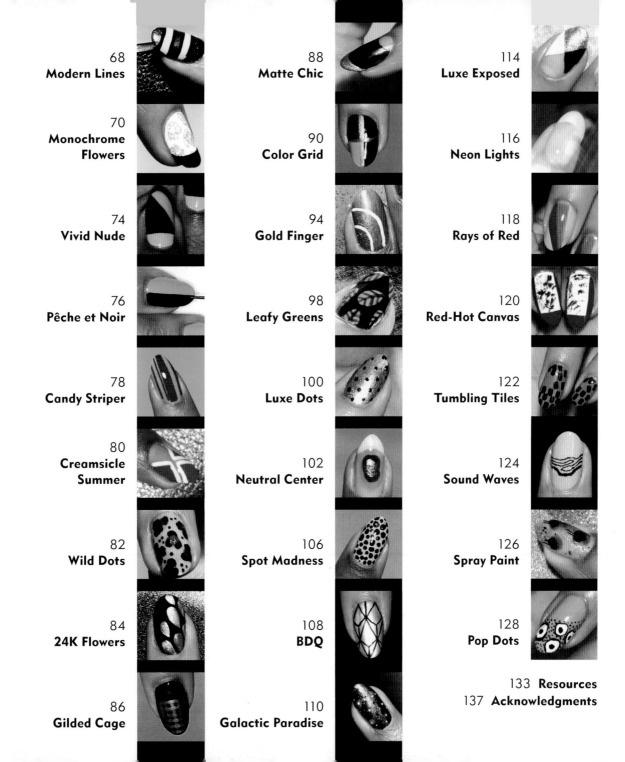

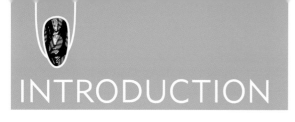

INTRODUCTION

Art has always been a part of my life, and so have manicures. I was in junior high school when I first did my own nails—I distinctly remember the metallic red polish I used. Soon I was heading to the drugstore to buy press-on nails, which I cut, filed, and shaped the way I liked. As time went on, my nail designs became more elaborate and I began to treat manicures as another form of artistic expression long before it became a trend.

I have been training as an artist from middle school through college, but a few years ago I began following the work of other professional nail artists and was inspired to seek out a new direction. With my business partner Gabe Vega, I set up a blog, elsalonsito.com, and started posting my work. Through Gabe's efforts—and those of his creative management agency, EL Management—my following grew, and I began working with companies like

Revlon, Maybelline, and Essie. Soon, *Marie Claire* magazine featured me as one of their favorite bloggers.

Nails are like tiny canvases to me. I love decorating them with all kinds of intricate designs and details—something I don't do when creating art on a larger scale. I hope this book inspires and encourages your inner artist, too. The designs and techniques featured here will show you how easy it is to create something personal and special—whether it's an intricate design for your wedding day or an homage to someone loved and lost. Think of your nail art as another form of self-expression: it's body art that can be as intricate as a tattoo but infinitely more changeable.

I love geometric patterns and textile design. The artist Keith Haring's use of smooth, repetitive lines has been a huge influence on my work, as has the fashion design of

Alexander McQueen—in fact, one of my most popular nail designs (Spray Paint, described on page 126) was inspired by the McQueen exhibit *Savage Beauty* at the Metropolitan Museum of Art. Another source of ideas is the public library. I often go there to read books on art and fashion, sketching out my ideas in notebooks and then executing them on false nails that fill my portfolio.

Knowing how your nails work and how to care for them is like preparing a canvas for painting—you want the best surface on which to create your amazing art. So before you turn to the nail art tutorials, be sure to study the basic manicure section of this book first. Most of my clients prefer gel manicures, so that their designs will last for weeks on end. But even if you're a beginner, once you understand the art *behind* the polishing of a nail and learn proper nail care, your manicures can last more than a week, too.

Great nail art starts with a good manicure, but it's also the result of practice—before I was able to create the designs you see on these pages, I went through a lot of trial and error, and you will, too. But your efforts will result in beautiful designs—I promise!

Start with the basic designs and practice, practice, practice. Then move to the more intricate patterns without fear; after all, there's no right or wrong when it comes to nail art. Consider these designs an open platform for your own self-expression—I encourage you to change the colors, combine different elements, and take them even further to express your own style.

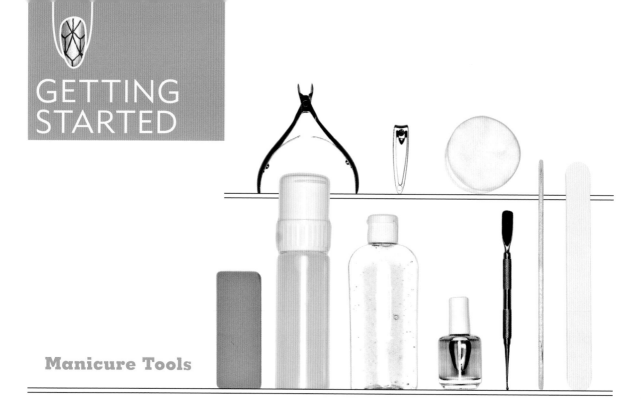

GETTING STARTED

Manicure Tools

- **Large paper towel or small hand towel to cover your work surface**
- **Nail polish remover**
- **Cotton pads**
- **Nail clippers**
- **100–180 grit nail file** for filing and shaping
- **240 grit buffer** to smooth the nail surface
- **Cuticle remover**
- **Metal cuticle pusher, or orangewood stick**
- **Cuticle nippers** (to be used with caution)

- **Nail plate primer** This solution, available at beauty stores, will remove any natural oils from your nail plate, which helps the polish adhere to your nail. You can also use isopropyl alcohol (70% or more by volume).
- **Base coat** This is a vital part of any manicure. Not only will it help prevent nail polish from staining your natural nails, it also serves as a glue that grabs the polish and holds it on your nails.

- **Top coat** Essential for a smooth, finished look and to protect your design.
- **Matte-finish top coat** This can give a special effect to a basic, one-color manicure or add an extra element to a nail art design.
- **Quick-dry solution** I prefer to let nails dry naturally, but for those occasions when you're in a hurry, you can use a quick-dry solution. This comes in spray form or drops, or as a brush-on oil.

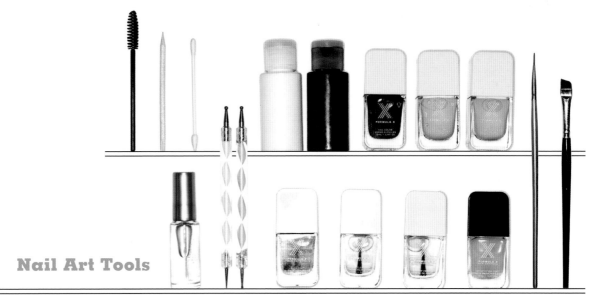

Nail Art Tools

Makeup cotton swabs
Cotton swabs with pointed tips are great for cleaning around the nail if you get polish on your skin. Just dip it in a bit of nail polish remover.

Aluminum foil Small squares of foil can serve as a palette for polish or paint that you'll be using in your designs.

Fine art brush I use thin brushes in various sizes and lengths for painting fine details on the nail. They are called "striping" brushes in beauty stores; I prefer brushes meant for oil paint, as they hold polish better and can be cleaned between colors with nail polish remover.

Angled brow brush This is my favorite way to clean nail polish from the surrounding skin. The angled brush gets into tight or hard-to-reach places.

Disposable mascara brush Another great tool for cleaning stubborn polish off your skin and from under your nail. Soak it in a bit of nail polish remover.

Dotting tool Made specifically for nail art, these tools are now widely available at drugstores and beauty stores, but a bobby pin or the head of a needle will work in a pinch (just be sure to cover the sharp end of the needle). The dotting tool should have both a small and a slightly larger head for making all sizes of dots.

Glow-in-the-dark top coat
An essential element of Neon Lights on page 116, this is a fun product that also allows secret "designs within a design" that are visible only in the dark or under UV light.

YOUR POLISH PALETTE

The selection of nail polish colors is more varied than ever before, and each visit to the drugstore or nail salon can make you feel like a kid in a candy store. Approach it like an artist. It's good to have primary and secondary colors on hand: blue, red, yellow, orange, purple, and green, as well as white and black. Beyond these, choose whatever shades inspire you.

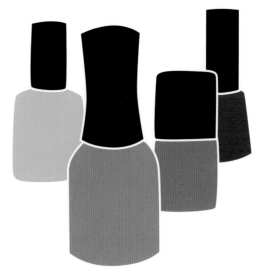

Sheer Polishes

Sheer polishes are great for creating layered looks and will help you accomplish ombre effects with ease. You can also use sheers to add shadows and depth to your design, just as a painter would with watered-down paint. When using a sheer polish next to an opaque polish, always apply the sheer polish first, then brush the opaque color over the sheer.

Opaque Polishes

Opaque polishes are perfect for design work because of their opacity. You'll use these to create sharp lines and details.

Glittery Polishes

Glittery polishes definitely add something extra to your nails. There are a variety of glitters, from fine (sandlike) glitter to chunky flakes where you can clearly see the individual pieces. All of them bring some bling to the nail, but each has its own unique characteristics as well.

Acrylic Paint

Acrylic paint doesn't dry out as quickly as nail polish, which is helpful when you lay out your color palette for nail art. It's great for painting super-fine details; while nail polish is naturally thick and fast drying, acrylic paint is very fluid, enabling you to draw much finer lines. You can find it in any craft store—look for the fluid type, not the more common thick, gel-like paint. I have all the primary and secondary colors mentioned earlier in acrylic paint as well as polish, but I find myself using black and white acrylic for detailing.

AMI'S BASIC MANICURE

TAKE YOUR TIME

Set aside enough time to complete your manicure without rushing. One of the simple keys to a good-looking, long-lasting manicure is allowing enough drying time between steps and at the finish. Go slowly and there's less chance for mistakes.

SET UP YOUR SPACE

Find a spot in your house where you can get a little messy—even if you're careful, you don't want to be working near a white rug or light-colored furniture. Pick a space with good ventilation, either in a large, open room or near an opened window. Lay down newspaper, paper towels, or a small hand towel to protect your work surface. Separate your tools, placing manicure tools (files, clippers) to one side and nail art tools (brushes, dotting tools) to the other.

PREP YOUR POLISH

Most of us are accustomed to shaking the bottle of nail polish before we unscrew the cap. The problem is, shaking creates air pockets in the polish, which transfer to your nail surface as you paint and leave you with bubbles instead of a smooth surface. To prevent bubbling, always roll the bottle between your hands until the color looks even throughout.

THE DRY MANICURE, STEP BY STEP

What's a dry manicure? A dry manicure is one in which you do not soak your hands in any water prior to working on your nails. That's right—I recommend that you don't soak your nails. Your manicure will last longer and here's why: your nails are porous, so if you soak them, they absorb water and expand—and they will not dry in the time it takes for you to prep your nails for polish. As they dry and shrink back to their natural shape, the polish will shift and crack. It's more important to clean the nail plate with primer or alcohol. Stay away from water.

- Remove old nail polish with a cotton pad soaked in remover.

- If your nails are exceptionally long or very hard, use clippers to cut them back before filing.

- File your nails to the desired shape. Always file to the center from both sides, meaning from each outer edge to the middle of the nail. Don't saw the file back and forth; it weakens the nail.

- Buff your nail plate to create a smooth surface. Gently go over the entire nail with the buffer, always moving from the base to the tip. Your polish will be smoother and shine more.

- Push back your cuticles. Apply a mild cuticle remover (gel hand sanitizer works well for this) and push back gently with a metal cuticle pusher or an orangewood stick. *Never* cut your cuticles.

- Wipe the nail plate clean with a primer or alcohol.

- Apply a thin base coat. Make sure to cover the entire nail. The base coat dries quickly, so there's no need to wait before moving on to the next step.

- Apply polish, working from the pinkie to the thumb, and starting on your dominant hand. Start to polish in the center of the nail and brush toward the tip. Then fill in on either side of the nail. Don't forget to "cap off" the nail by painting across the tip—this will help your manicure last longer. Repeat with a second coat.

- Allow the polish to dry for two to three minutes before applying the top coat. Always remember to cap off each nail, as this helps seal in your color and design.

Always complete the basic manicure before beginning your nail art.

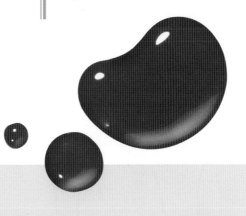

CORRECTING MISTAKES

If you get nail polish on the skin around the nail, lightly dip an angled eyebrow brush in nail polish remover.

If you nick the surface of the nail in the middle of your paint job, dip the angled eyebrow brush in nail polish remover and lightly brush over the nicked area. You can also dip your finger in nail polish remover and lightly tap the area to smooth it before you go over it with another layer of color.

AMI'S TOP TIPS FOR NAIL ART

Choose Your Nail Shape

I don't think there's a "right" shape for any nail. Choose what works for you and what complements your nail design.

Round. A shorter nail that's very easy to maintain, this shape is especially attractive if you have a longer nail bed.

Oval. This is a classic nail shape that looks good on everyone. It allows for more length while still appearing graceful.

Square. This is a great shape for shorter nails.

Squoval. Probably the most popular nail shape, because it offers the elegance of the oval shape with the strength of the square.

Almond. The most dramatic nail shape, it makes a strong fashion statement.

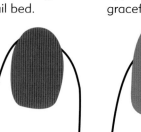

SUCCESS

[Practice, practice, practice!

[Less is more. To create fine lines with acrylic paint, use less paint on the brush. To create fine lines with nail polish, make sure the polish is fresh and don't oversaturate your nail-striping brush with polish.

[Always paint your dominant hand first. It's much harder to paint after you've painted the nondominant hand.

Ami's Top Tips for Making Your Manicure Last

Prepping your nails is vital to a long-lasting manicure.	Don't soak. Always do a dry manicure.	Clean the surface of your nail plate with primer before applying polish to help with adhesion.	Always cap off the nail to seal in the color and design.	If need be, apply a thin layer of top coat every three days or so. This will help keep your nails shiny and lengthen the life of your mani.

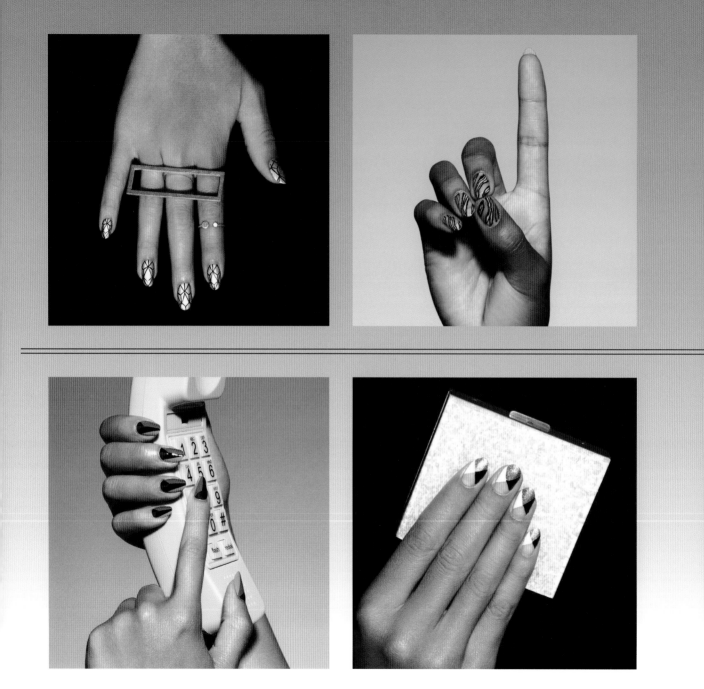

───── NAIL ART

BABY LEOPARD

Take a walk on the wild side with this fashionable animal print.

Tools

- ¬ **Base coat**
- ¬ **Pale yellow polish**
- ¬ **Shimmery nude polish**
- ¬ **Darker nude polish**
- ¬ **Dotting tool or toothpick**
- ¬ **Black polish or acrylic paint**
- ¬ **Top coat**

1. Apply two coats of pale yellow polish and let dry for two minutes. Working from the cuticle up, paint one coat of shimmery nude polish halfway up the nail. Let dry for two minutes.

2. Again working from the cuticle up, paint one coat of darker nude polish, stopping a bit before the edge of the shimmery nude polish. Let dry for two minutes.

3. Using the smaller end of the dotting tool and working from the cuticle to the tip, create the leopard spots by painting broken circles with black polish. The spots should be very abstract, so don't worry about making them perfect. Let dry for two minutes, then seal the design with top coat.

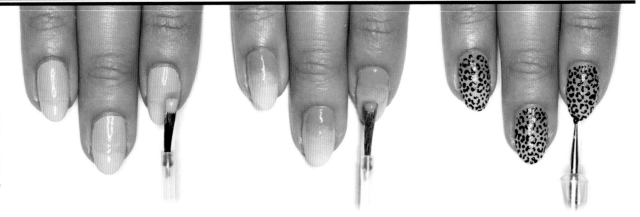

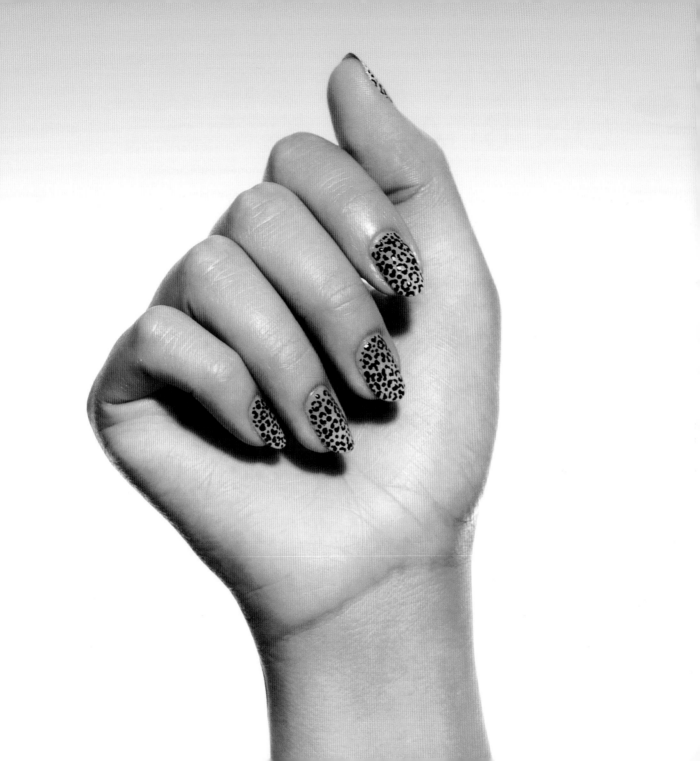

BLACK ON BLACK

A combination of sheer and opaque black polish, this design is subtle yet über sophisticated. Use acrylic paint to create the very thin lines and another shade of black for the thick V.

Tools

- Base coat
- Sheer black polish
- Fine art brush
- Black acrylic paint
- Opaque black polish
- Top coat

1. Apply one thin and very sheer coat of sheer black polish. Let dry for one minute.

2. With a fine art brush and black acrylic paint, make a large X in thin lines across the entire nail. Continuing to keep the lines thin, outline the X three more times.

3. With a fine art brush and opaque black polish, paint a thick V at the top and the base of the nail, with the points connecting at the center. Let dry for two minutes, then seal the design with top coat.

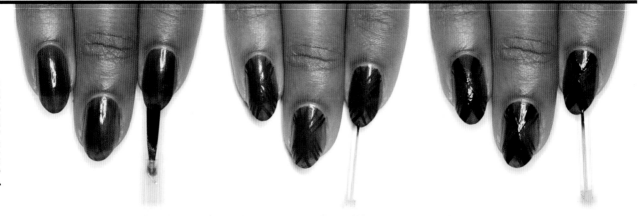

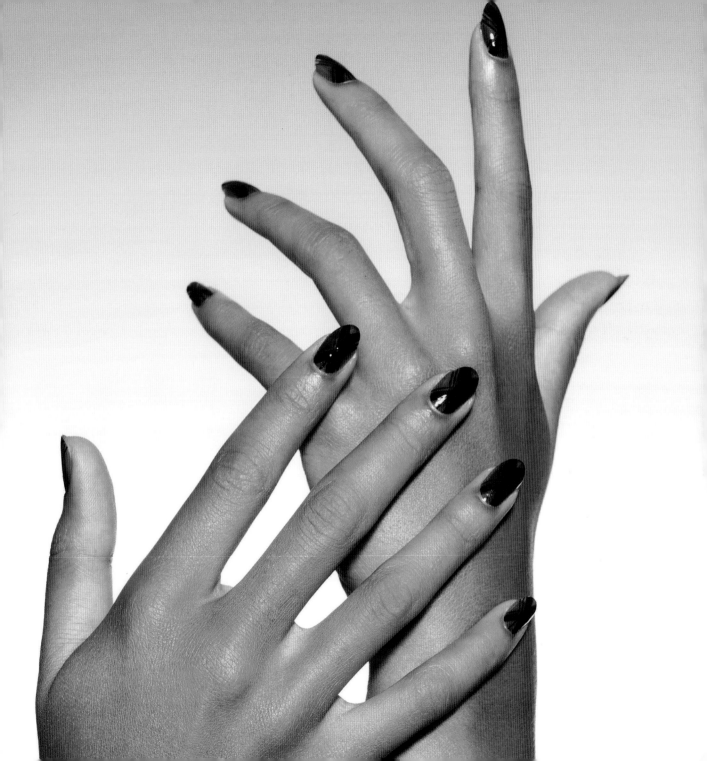

BLACK MATTE SNAKESKIN

Sophisticated and sexy, this look gives a positively reptilian impression.

Tools

⌐ **Base coat**

⌐ **Opaque black polish or acrylic paint**

⌐ **Matte-finish top coat**

⌐ **Red polish with fine glitter**

⌐ **Bright red polish**

⌐ **Top coat**

1. Apply two coats of opaque black polish and let dry for two minutes.

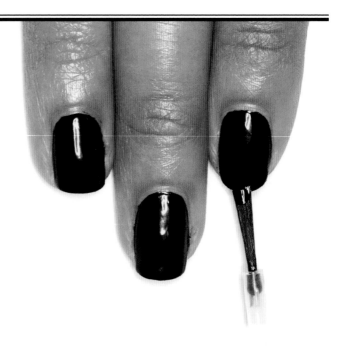

2. Paint matte-finish top coat over the entire nail and let dry for two minutes.

3. Wipe most of the opaque black polish off its brush, then paint diamond shapes randomly across the nail, leaving space in between the shapes.

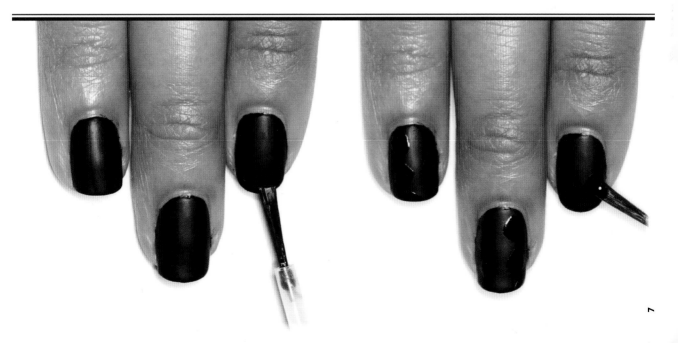

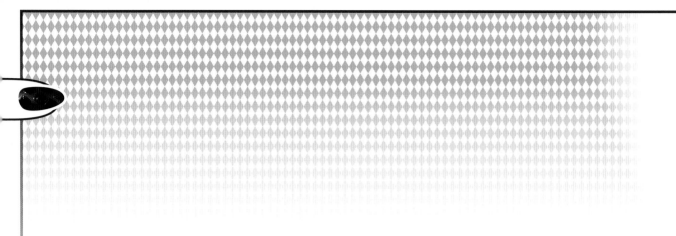

4. Repeat Step 3 with red polish with fine glitter.

5. Repeat Step 3 with bright red polish. Apply regular top coat on the diamond shapes only, to add extra dimension to the design.

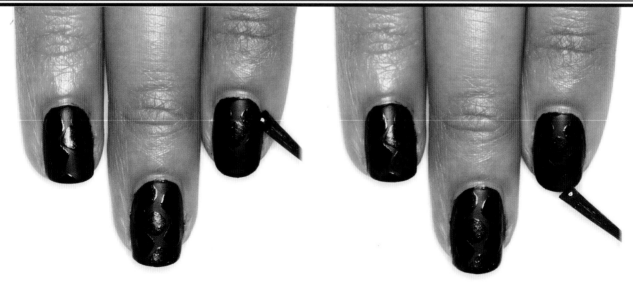

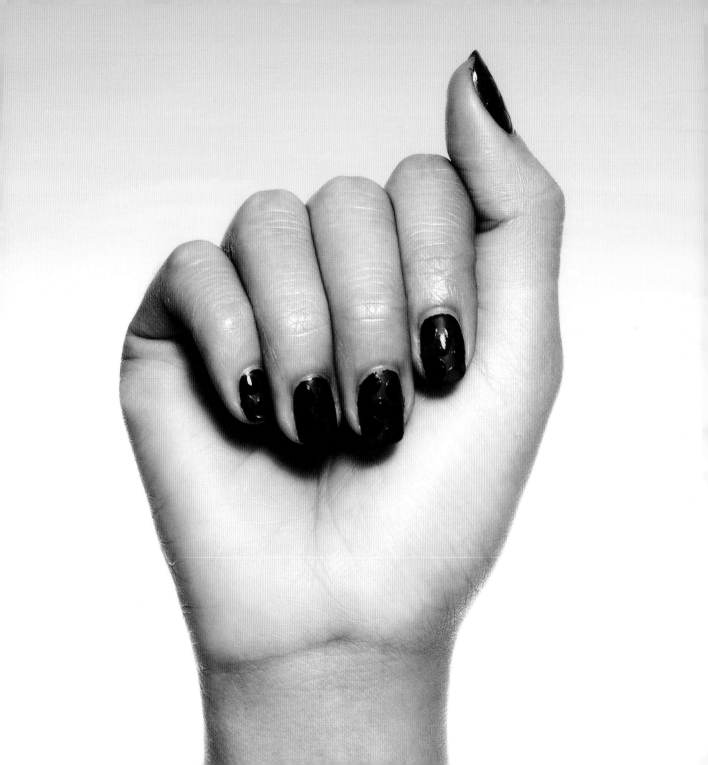

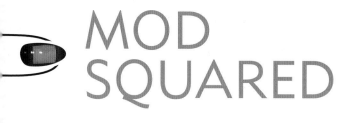

MOD SQUARED

An elegant combination of simple shapes painted in jewel-like colors, this design is a perfect partner for your fall wardrobe or anytime you want a dramatic look.

Tools

⌐ **Base coat**

⌐ **Dark blue polish**

⌐ **Bright orange polish**

⌐ **Fine art brush**

⌐ **Bright red polish**

⌐ **Top coat**

1. Apply two coats of dark blue polish and let dry for two minutes.

2. Paint a rectangle of bright orange polish in the center of the nail. Don't worry about perfect edges, but do leave some room on all sides. Let dry for one minute.

3. Using a fine art brush and bright red polish, outline the orange rectangle with a wide border. Let dry for two minutes, then seal the design with top coat.

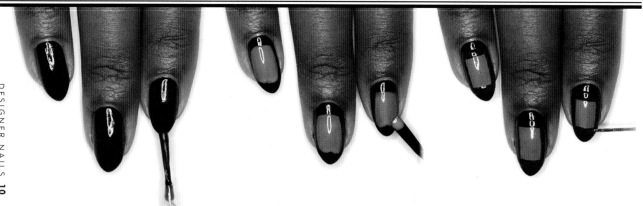

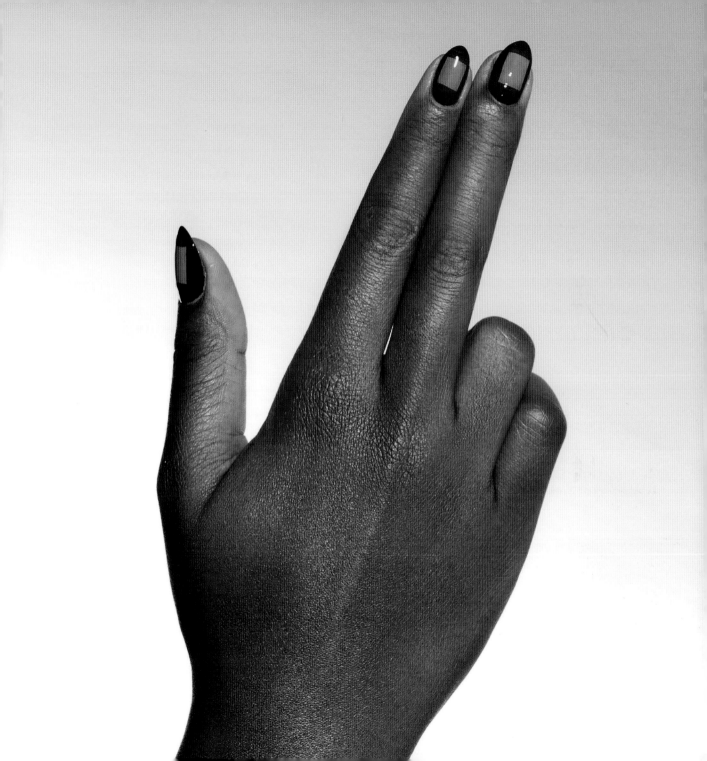

BADGE OF GOLD

This is a simple yet elegant design that features a subtle chevron of gold polish at the nail base.

Tools

- Base coat
- Creamy soft yellow polish
- Fine art brush
- Metallic gold polish
- Top coat

1. Apply two coats of creamy soft yellow polish and let dry for two minutes.

2. Create an elongated triangle or pyramid shape at the base of the nail with a fine art brush and metallic gold polish. With the tip of the brush, mark the top of the pyramid at the center of the nail, then connect it to the base with adjoining lines before filling in the triangle. Let dry for two minutes, then seal the design with top coat.

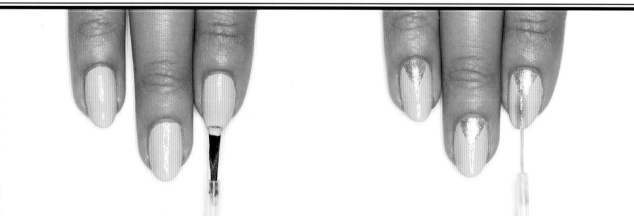

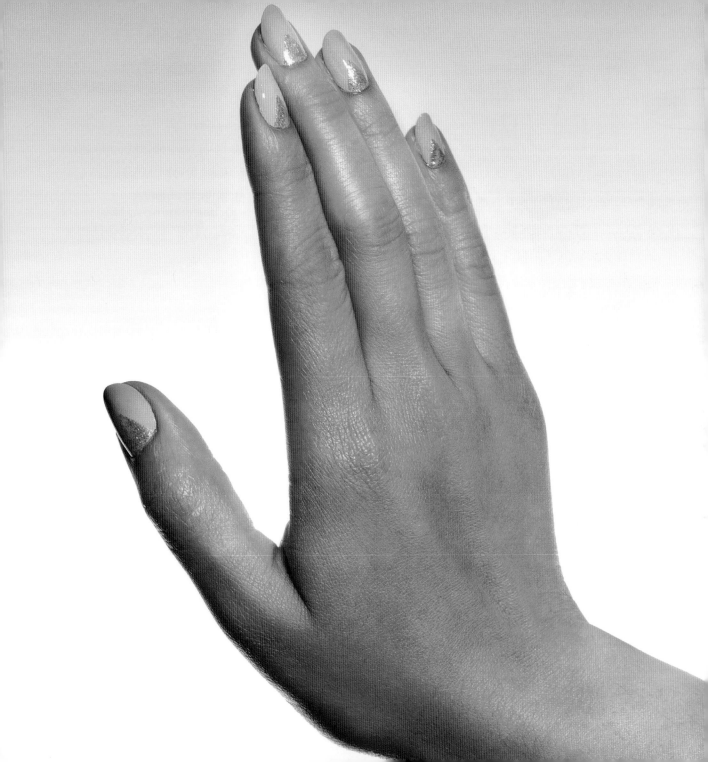

TRUE BLUE

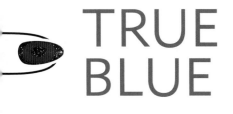

These dual shades of blue shimmer like deep pools of water reflecting the night sky.

Tools

- Base coat
- Medium blue polish
- Fine art brush
- Metallic blue polish with fine glitter
- Top coat

1. Apply two coats of medium blue polish and let dry for two minutes.

2. With a fine art brush, paint a small oval of metallic blue polish with fine glitter in the center of the nail.

3. With a fine art brush, outline the entire nail with a larger oval of metallic blue polish with fine glitter, creating a bull's-eye pattern. Let dry for two minutes, then seal the design with top coat.

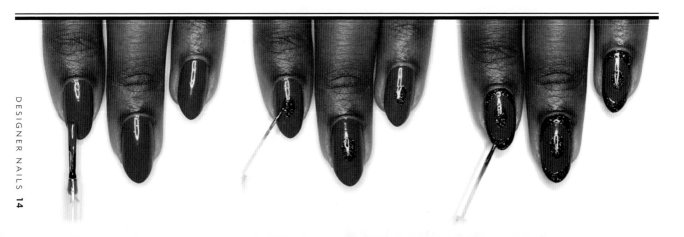

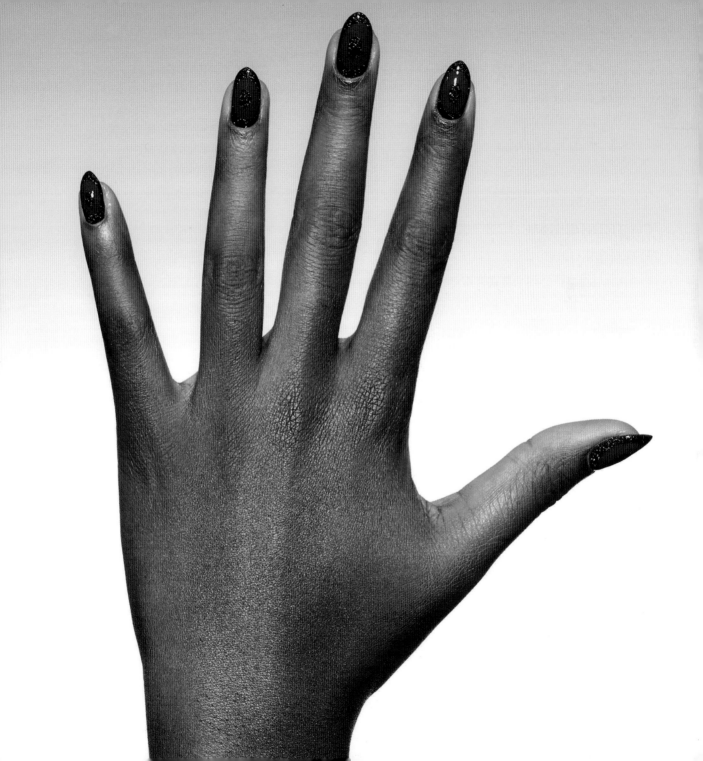

GILDED MOON

The black moon gives this design a touch of added drama, but use any dark, rich color that inspires you here.

Tools

- ◻ **Base coat**
- ◻ **Sheer polish with fine gold glitter**
- ◻ **Metallic gold polish with fine glitter**
- ◻ **Fine art brush**
- ◻ **Black polish or acrylic paint**
- ◻ **Top coat**

1. Wipe most of the sheer polish with fine gold glitter off its brush, then dab it all over the nail. Leave some exposed spaces on the nail.

2. Repeat Step 1 with metallic gold polish with fine glitter. Fill in some of the open spaces, but leave some of the nail exposed.

3. With a fine art brush and black polish, outline the cuticle of the nail. Outline the curved top of the half moon and then fill in the crescent. Let dry for two minutes, then seal the design with top coat.

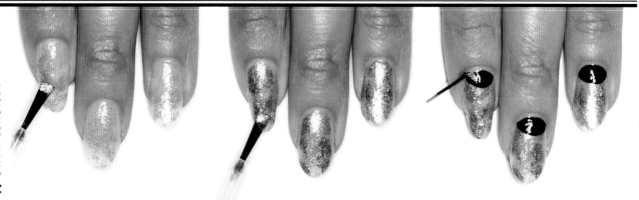

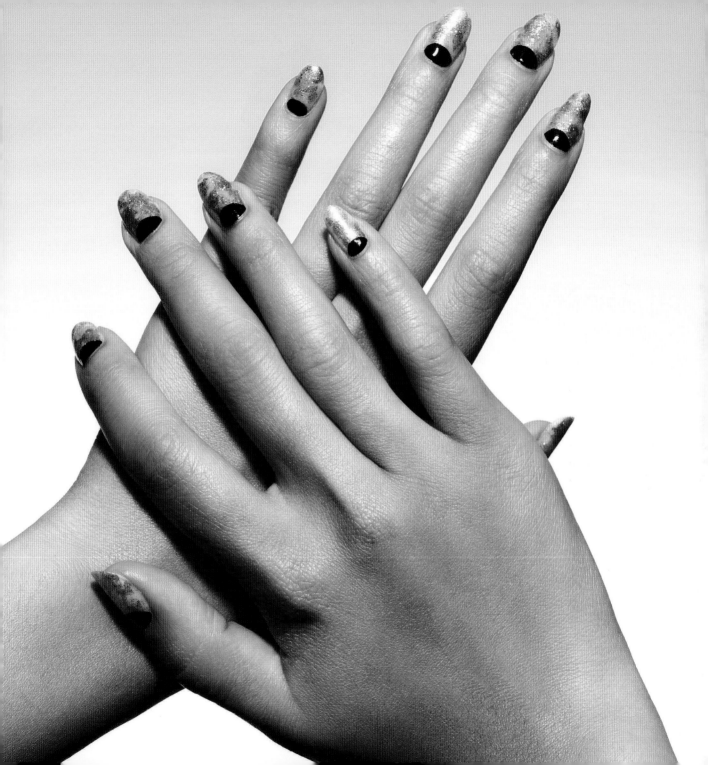

MOON GLOW

Miami modern meets extraterrestrial style in this otherworldly design.

Tools

⌐ **Base coat**

⌐ **Rich pastel orange polish**

⌐ **Fine art brush**

⌐ **Bright pale blue polish**

⌐ **Opaque white polish or acrylic paint**

⌐ **Top coat**

1. Apply two coats of rich pastel orange polish and let dry for two minutes.

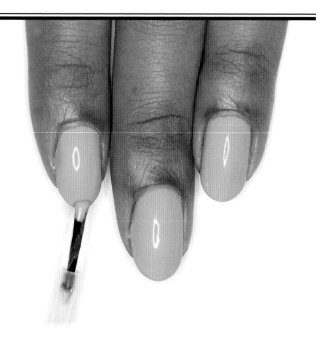

2. With a fine art brush and bright pale blue polish, paint a half moon at the base of the nail. Trace the cuticle area first, then draw the top curved line and fill in the open space. Let dry for two minutes.

3. With a fine art brush and opaque white polish, trace the top arc of the blue half moon, then paint a line straight from the center of the half moon to the tip of the nail.

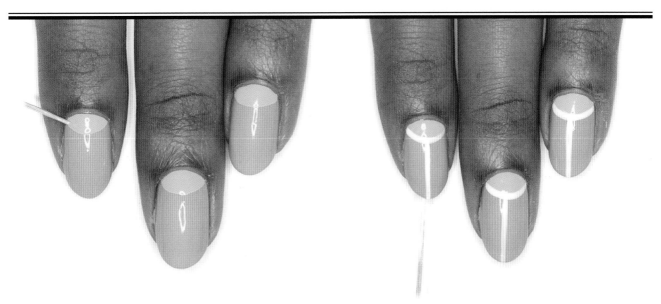

4. Bring the brush back down from the tip, curving the brush outward and over the side of the half moon. Repeat on the other side and fill in any space left unpainted by the white. Let dry for two minutes, then seal the design with top coat.

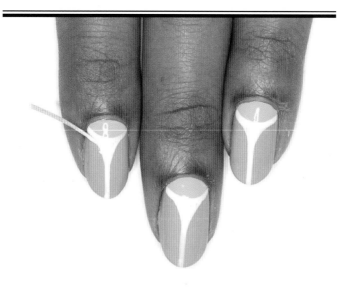

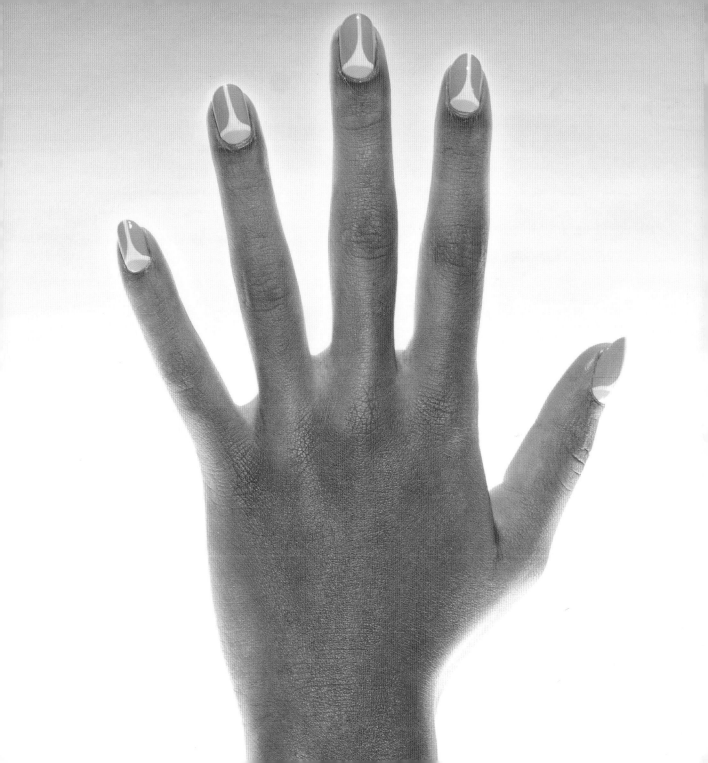

POP NEONS

Fun and funky! Take your pick of bright neon shades to bring this design to life.

Tools

- ⊓ **Base coat**
- ⊓ **Black polish or acrylic paint**
- ⊓ **Fine art brush**
- ⊓ **Pale blue neon polish**
- ⊓ **Yellow neon polish**
- ⊓ **Purple neon polish**
- ⊓ **Top coat**

1. Paint a line of black polish diagonally across the nail. Begin at one edge of the moon and end at the edge of the finger, where the nail tip begins. Fill in the area above the line with black polish and let dry for two minutes.

2. With a fine art brush, paint triangle shapes of various sizes randomly across the nail with pale blue, yellow neon, and purple neon polishes. Let dry for two minutes, then seal the design with top coat.

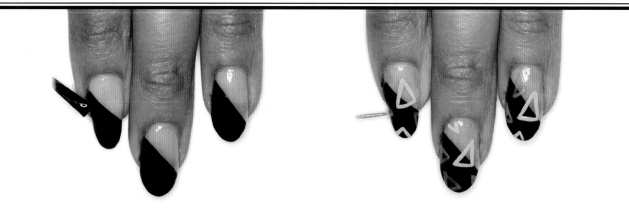

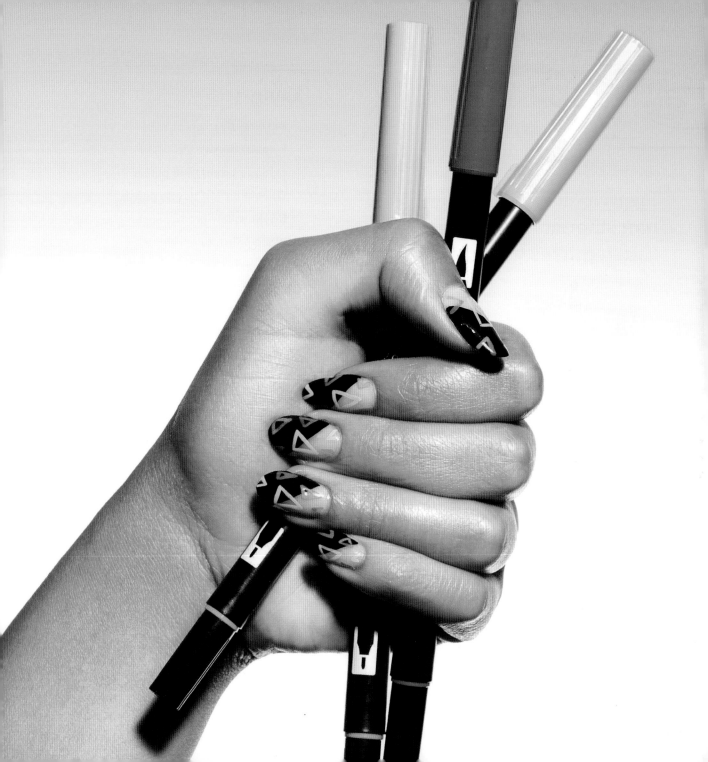

PASTEL WAVES

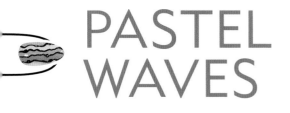

Pretty pastels with downtown chic; the black outlining really makes the colors pop.

Tools

- ¬ **Base coat**
- ¬ **Fine art brush**
- ¬ **Opaque bright pink polish**
- ¬ **Opaque bright purple polish**
- ¬ **Bright yellow-green polish**
- ¬ **Black polish or acrylic paint**
- ¬ **Top coat**

1. With a fine art brush, paint a squiggly line of opaque bright pink polish down the center of the nail.

2. Repeat Step 1, first painting an opaque bright purple and then a bright yellow-green squiggly line on either side of the pink line. Don't worry if there are gaps between the lines. Let dry for two minutes.

3. With a fine art brush and black polish, outline all three colors. As you paint, add the occasional small swirl to the lines. Let dry for two minutes, then seal the design with top coat.

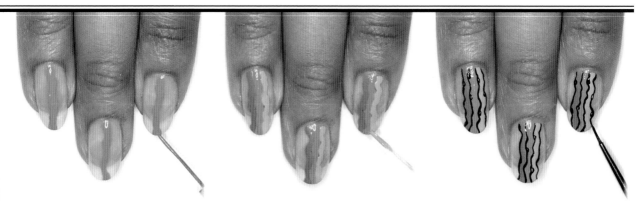

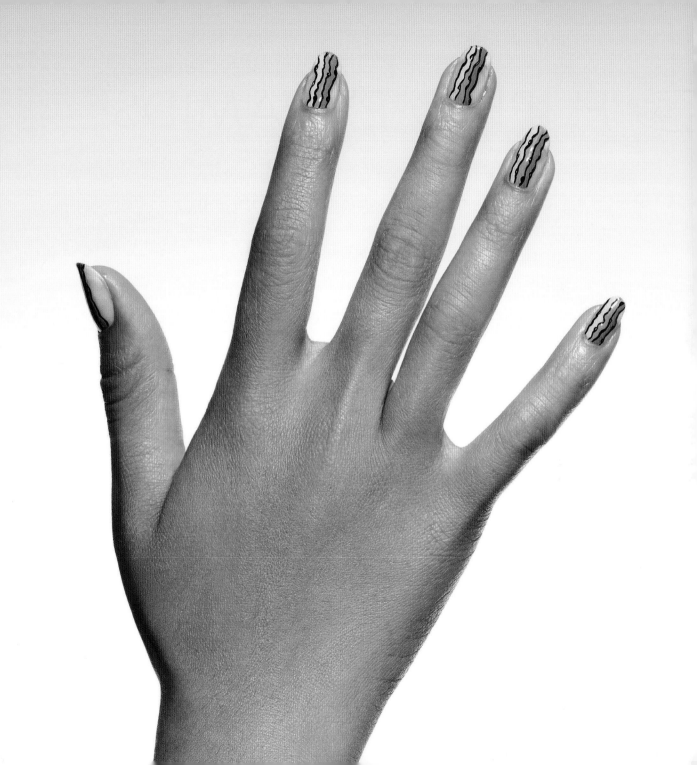

FLIPPED PYRAMIDS

A super graphic design in black and white, this would be just as dramatic in any two coordinating colors. For fine details like these, I find acrylic paint easier to work with than polish.

Tools

- ¬ **Base coat**
- ¬ **Opaque white acrylic paint**
- ¬ **Black polish or acrylic paint**
- ¬ **Small fine art brush**
- ¬ **Top coat**

1. Working from the cuticle to the tip, paint one half of the nail with opaque white polish.

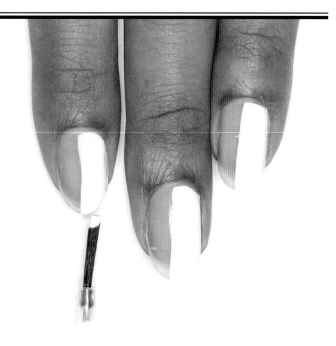

2. Working from the cuticle to the tip, paint the other half of the nail with black polish. Let dry for two minutes.

3. With a small fine art brush and black acrylic paint, paint small black triangles on the white half of the nail. Sharpen the edges of the triangles by tracing their outlines with white.

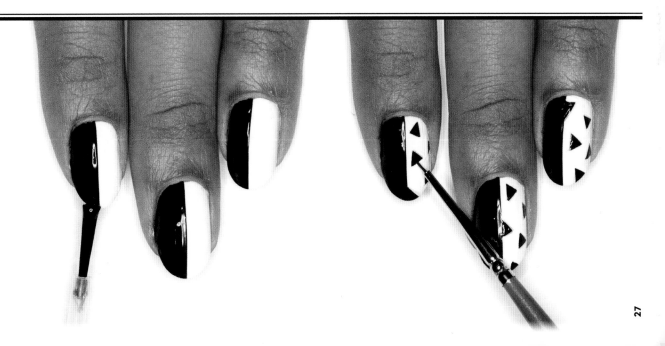

4. Repeat Step 3 on the black half of the nail with opaque white acrylic paint. Sharpen the triangle edges by tracing their outlines with black. Let dry for two minutes, then seal the design with top coat.

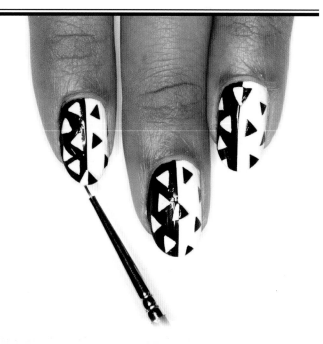

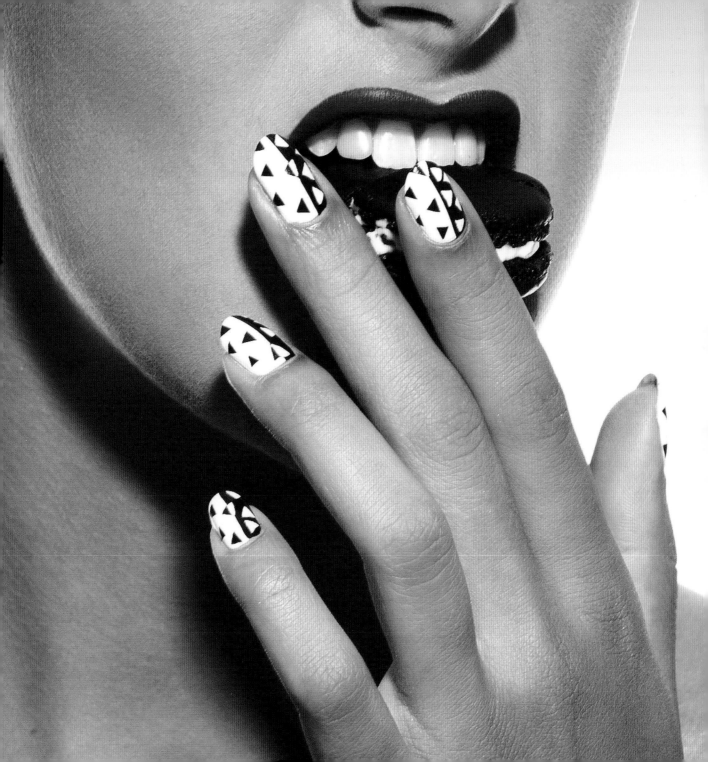

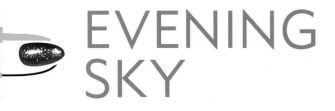

EVENING SKY

This design makes me think of the sky in early evening, when shades of blue turn to dark and the stars are just beginning to twinkle.

Tools

¬ **Base coat**

¬ **Opaque light blue polish**

¬ **Dark blue polish**

¬ **Sheer dark blue polish with fine glitter**

¬ **Top coat**

1. Apply one coat of opaque light blue polish and let dry for two minutes.

2. Paint a second coat of opaque light blue polish on only one half of the nail, then quickly paint the other half with dark blue polish, overlapping on the light side and blending the two as you go. Let dry for two minutes.

3. Beginning on the darker side, paint a heavy coat of sheer dark blue polish with fine glitter, brushing lighter as you move to the lighter side of the nail. Let dry for two minutes, then seal the design with top coat.

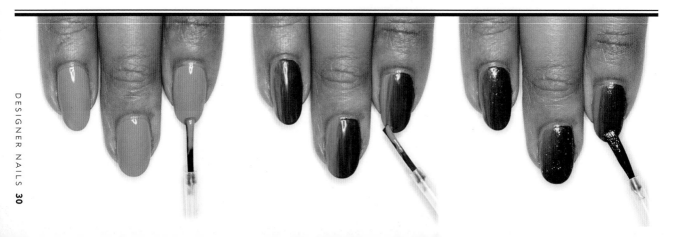

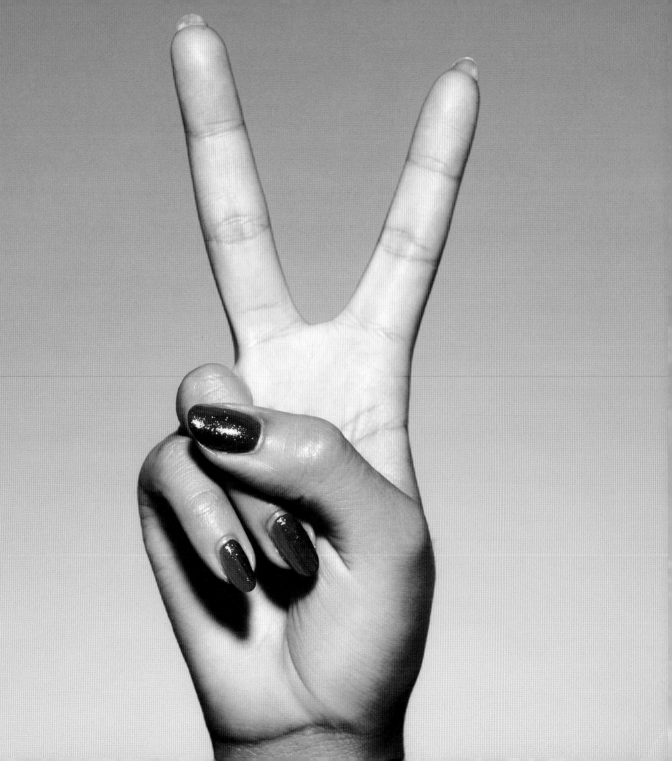

CLASSIC BLACK AND WHITE

A look that goes with everything, this is another design that will work well with lots of different color combinations.

Tools

□ **Base coat**

□ **Opaque white polish or acrylic paint**

□ **Fine art brush**

□ **Opaque black polish or acrylic paint**

□ **Top coat**

1. Apply two coats of opaque white polish and let dry for two minutes.

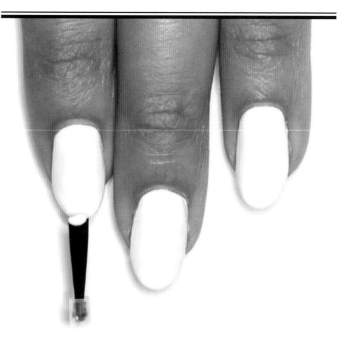

2. With a fine art brush and opaque black polish, paint a thin line diagonally across the nail. Start the line at one edge of the moon and end at the edge of the finger where the nail tip begins. Let dry for one minute.

3. Now paint thin vertical lines, working from cuticle to tip, leaving a generous amount of space between the lines.

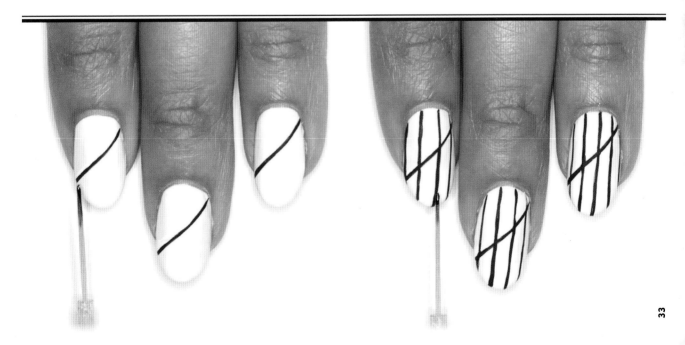

4. Fill in the space between the lines with opaque black polish, alternating the placement from top to bottom. Let dry for two minutes, then seal the design with top coat.

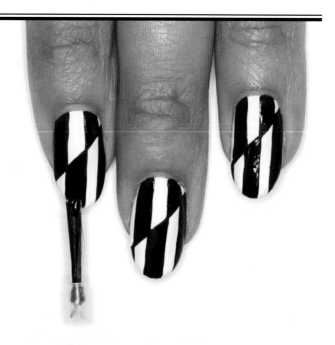

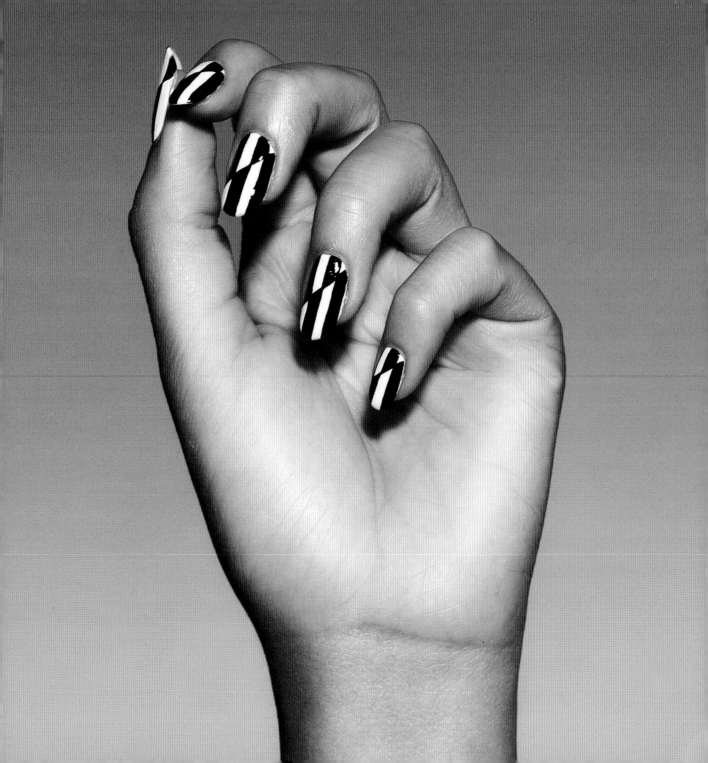

BRUSH STROKES

Another design that can appear in any number of color combinations, this is the simplest expression of the nail as canvas.

1. Apply two coats of dark purple polish and let dry for two minutes.

2. Wipe most of the bright green polish off its brush, then lightly stroke the remaining polish over the nail, barely touching the surface and creating random brushstrokes over the entire surface. Let dry for two minutes, then seal the design with top coat.

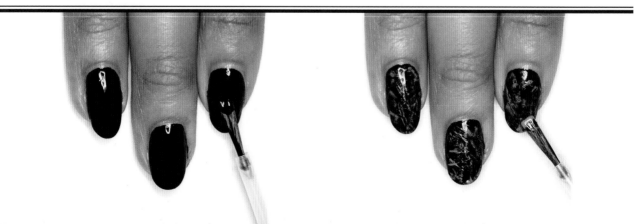

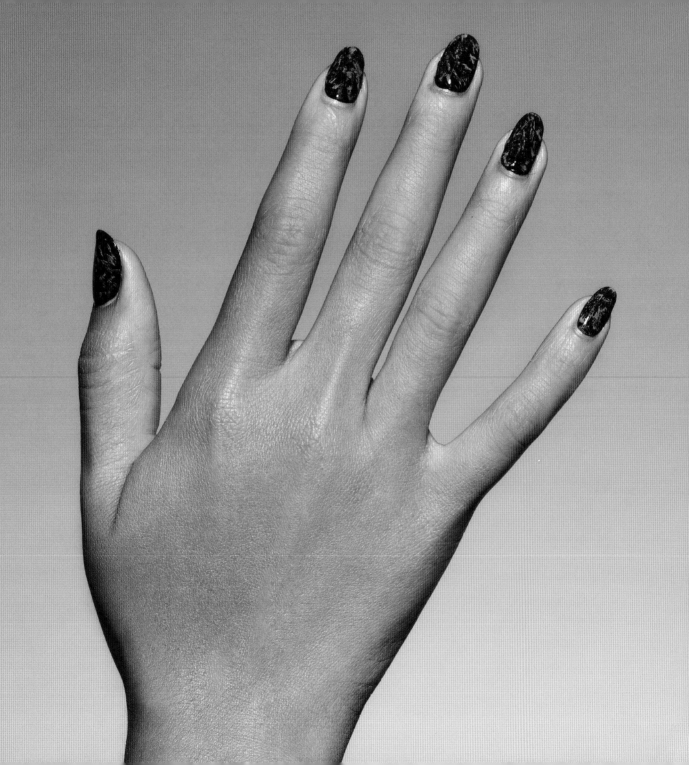

FRESH PRINTS

This design will definitely get some notice. I find acrylic paints work best with design details that are so small and that require such sharp edges.

Tools

- ☐ **Base coat**
- ☐ **Opaque white acrylic paint or polish**
- ☐ **Fine art brush**
- ☐ **Pale blue acrylic paint or polish**
- ☐ **Bright red acrylic paint or polish**
- ☐ **Bright yellow acrylic paint or polish**
- ☐ **Opaque black acrylic paint or polish**
- ☐ **Top coat**

1. Apply two coats of opaque white acrylic paint and let dry for two minutes.

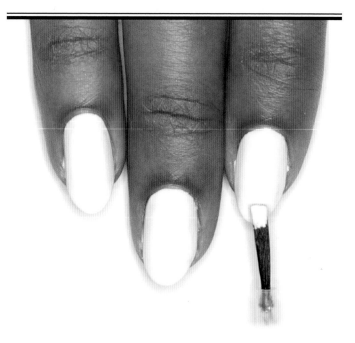

2. With a fine art brush and pale blue acrylic paint, paint randomly sized and spaced triangular shapes. Leave lots of space between the shapes.

3. Repeat Step 2 with bright red acrylic paint.

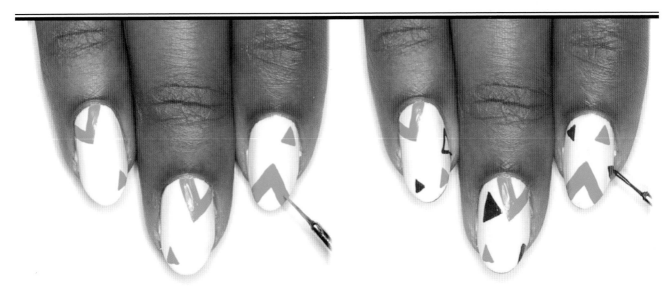

4. Add small triangles of bright yellow acrylic paint, then finish with opaque black acrylic paint, using it to fill in some of the triangles solidly or with horizontal and vertical lines. Let dry for two minutes, then seal the design with top coat.

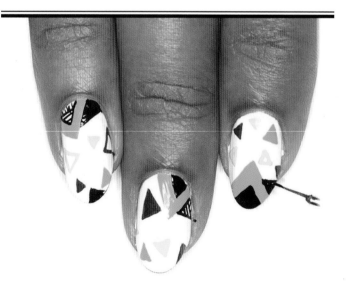

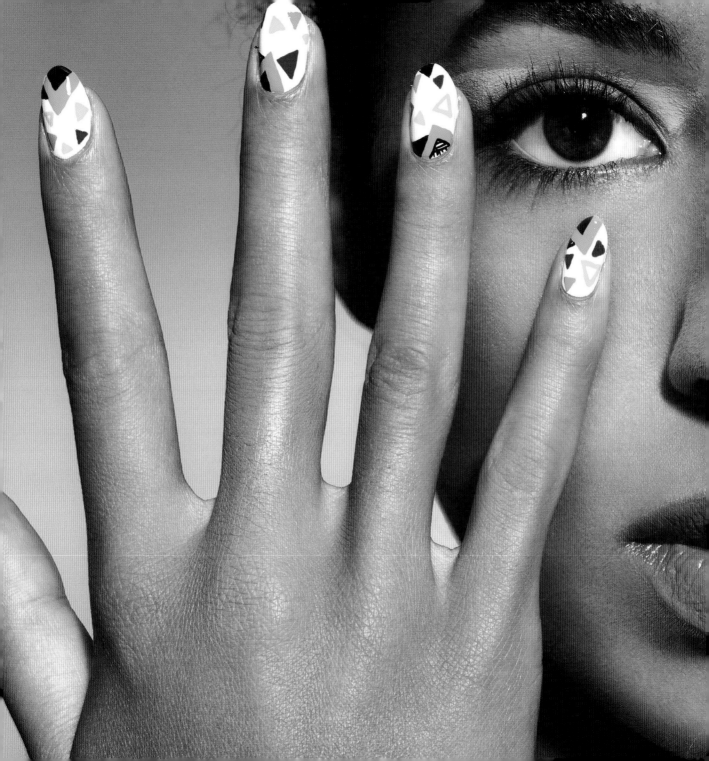

BERRY BLACK

Who says strawberries have to be red? Gray, black, white, and metallic add up to a design that will make people look twice. I like to use a fine art brush rather than a dotting tool for creating very tiny dots and irregular shapes such as these.

Tools

- ⌐ **Base coat**
- ⌐ **Light gray polish**
- ⌐ **Fine art brush**
- ⌐ **Opaque black polish or acrylic paint**
- ⌐ **Opaque white polish or acrylic paint**
- ⌐ **Metallic gold polish**
- ⌐ **Top coat**

1. Apply two coats of light gray polish and let dry for two minutes.

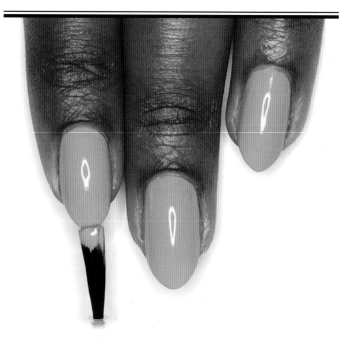

2. With a fine art brush and opaque black polish, paint a pattern of oval shapes across the entire nail. When placing the shapes, start from the center of the nail and work out toward the edges.

3. With a fine art brush and opaque white polish, paint very small white dots inside each oval.

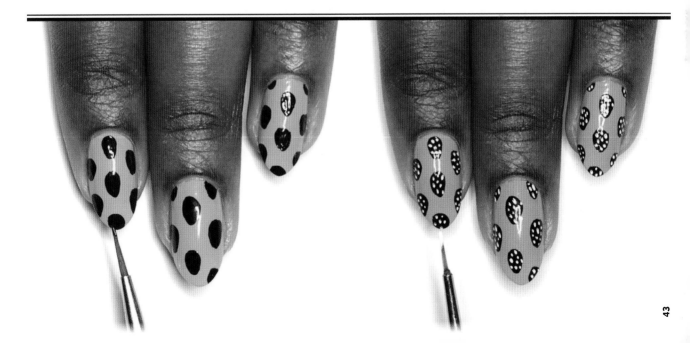

4. With a fine art brush and metallic gold polish, paint a cap of tiny leaves—four connected oval shapes—at the top of the ovals so they look like strawberries. Let dry for two minutes, then seal the design with top coat.

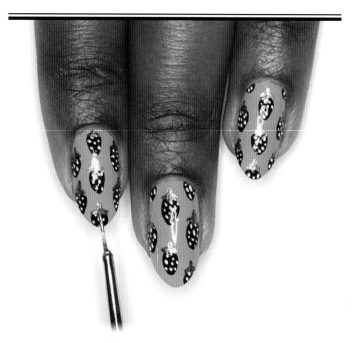

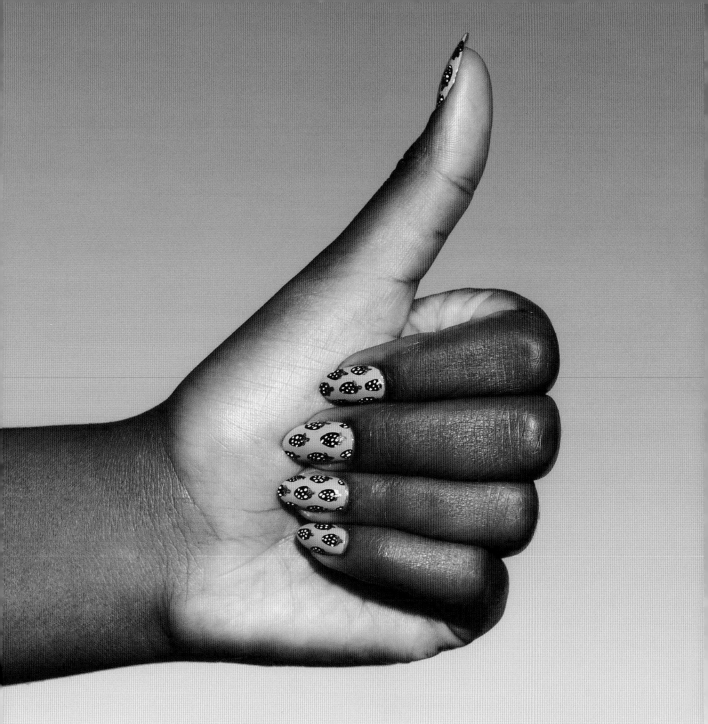

LEMON-LIME GEOMETRIC

Bright and fun, this design is a ray of sunshine, even on a rainy day.

Tools

- ¬ **Base coat**
- ¬ **Bright yellow polish**
- ¬ **Fine art brush**
- ¬ **Lime green polish**
- ¬ **Top coat**

1. Apply two coats of bright yellow polish and let dry for two minutes.

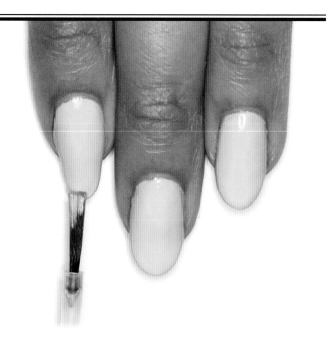

2. With a fine art brush, paint a thin line of lime green polish diagonally across the nail.

3. Starting from the end of the diagonal line, paint a lime green line across the top of the nail to make a triangle shape. Fill in the triangle with lime green polish.

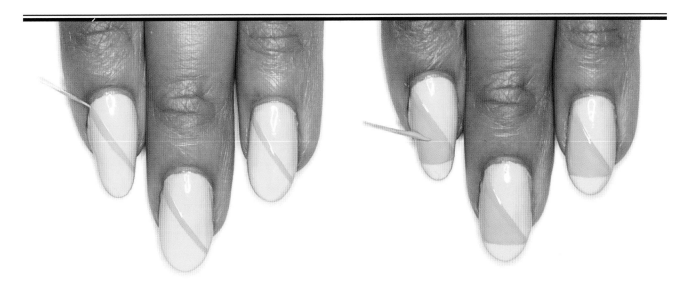

4. Working from the base point of the lime green triangle, paint a lime green line straight across the base of the nail. This forms a corresponding yellow triangle. Fill in the base of the nail with lime green polish. Let dry for two minutes, then seal the design with top coat.

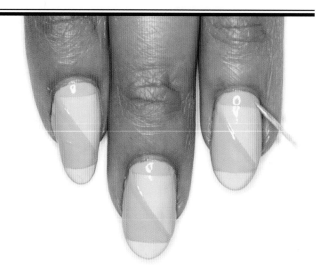

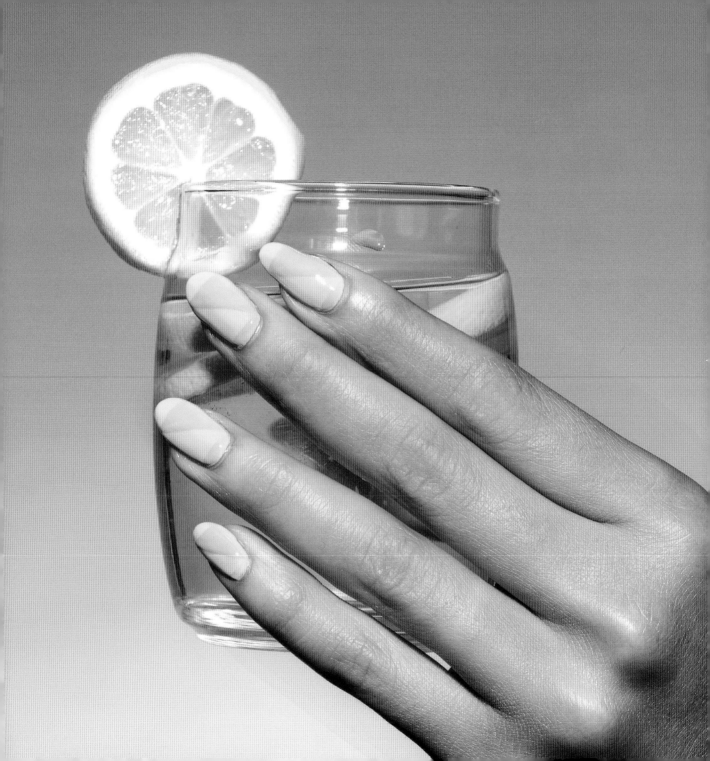

DECO LINES

Complementary shades of gold and olive green are the basis of a design reminiscent of the Art Deco period. Choose a gold metallic polish with green tones for the best result.

Tools

- ¬ **Base coat**
- ¬ **Fine art brush**
- ¬ **Gold metallic polish**
- ¬ **Olive green polish**
- ¬ **Top coat**

1. With a fine art brush and gold metallic polish, outline the top arc of the moon. Fill in the rest of the nail above, leaving the moon exposed. Let dry for two minutes.

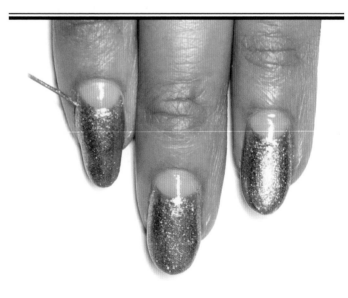

2. With a fine art brush and olive green polish, trace the top outline of the moon, then paint a line across the nail horizontally, almost at the very top of the nail.

3. Starting from the line painted at the top of the nail, mirror the arc of the half moon outline, but upside down. Paint a larger half circle, elongating the arc so that you meet the top of the half moon. If your nails are shorter than those shown here, you may want to paint fewer lines.

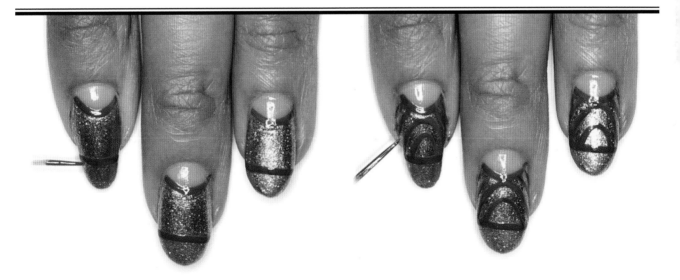

4. At the tip of the nail, use the olive green polish to paint vertical lines across the tip, above the original horizontal line. Let dry for two minutes, then seal the design with top coat.

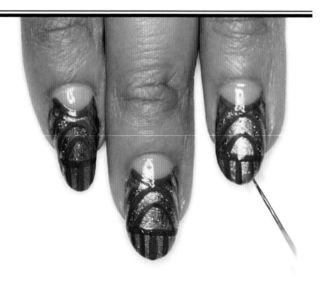

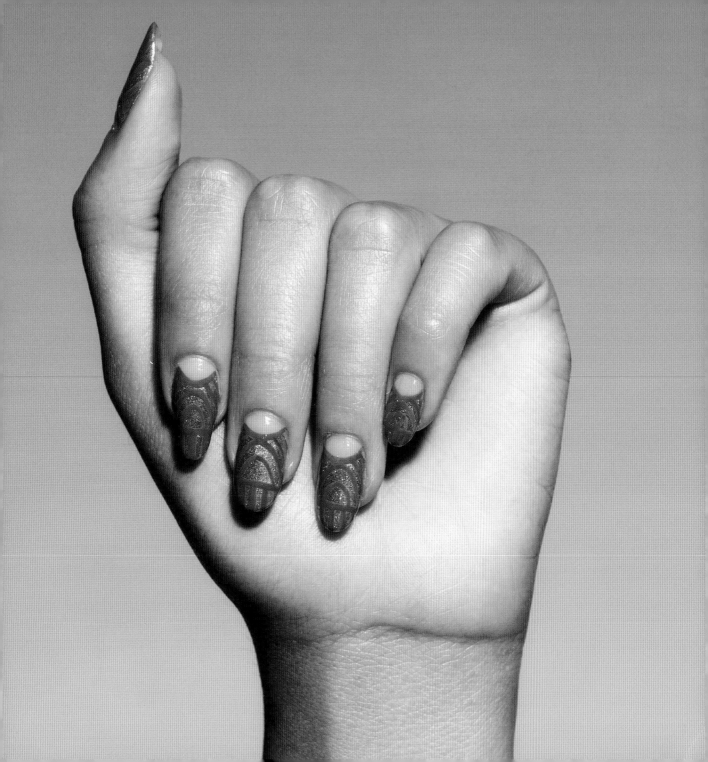

RETRO GEOMETRY

I was inspired to create this design by the bold geometric designs of contemporary art, especially the Cut-Outs of Henri Matisse.

Tools

- ⌐ **Base coat**
- ⌐ **Bright orange neon polish**
- ⌐ **Bright pink neon polish**
- ⌐ **Fine art brush**
- ⌐ **Sheer electric blue polish**
- ⌐ **Teal polish**
- ⌐ **Black polish or acrylic paint**
- ⌐ **Top coat**

1. Paint one half of the nail with bright orange neon polish, then paint the other half with bright pink neon polish. Let dry for two minutes.

2. With a fine art brush and sheer electric blue polish, paint a triangle at the base of the nail. One half of the triangle will appear black.

3. With a fine art brush and teal polish, paint a long, narrow triangle shape on the orange side of the nail, leaving the orange edge exposed. Repeat the same shape in black polish on the pink side, leaving the pink edge exposed. Let dry for two minutes, then seal the design with top coat.

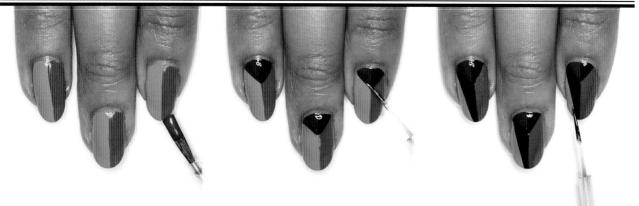

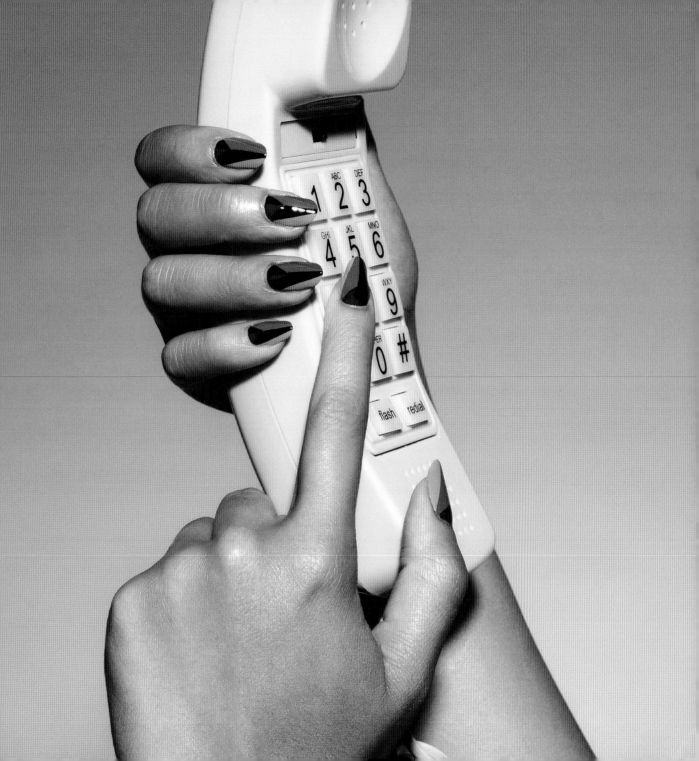

FLOWER PUDDLES

A pretty look for spring, or any time of year, this Impressionistic design resembles flower petals dotted with raindrops.

Tools

- ⌐ **Base coat**
- ⌐ **Opaque peach polish**
- ⌐ **Opaque coral polish**
- ⌐ **Pale blue polish**
- ⌐ **Pale purple polish**
- ⌐ **Lipstick brush**
- ⌐ **Nail polish remover**
- ⌐ **Top coat**

1. Using peach and coral polishes, apply random dots of each color over the nail. Dip a lipstick brush in nail polish remover and dab the center of each dot to pick up a bit of the color. Complete one or two fingers at a time; you don't want the polish to dry between steps.

2. Repeat Step 1 with the pale blue and pale purple polishes. Overlap some of the colors, but leave bare spaces in between the dots, too. Let dry for two minutes, then seal the design with top coat.

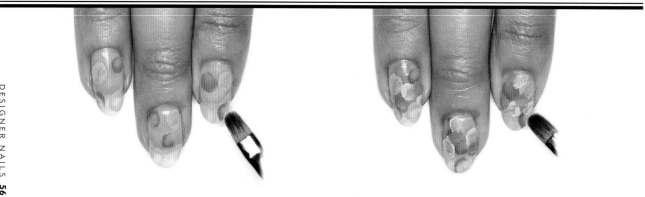

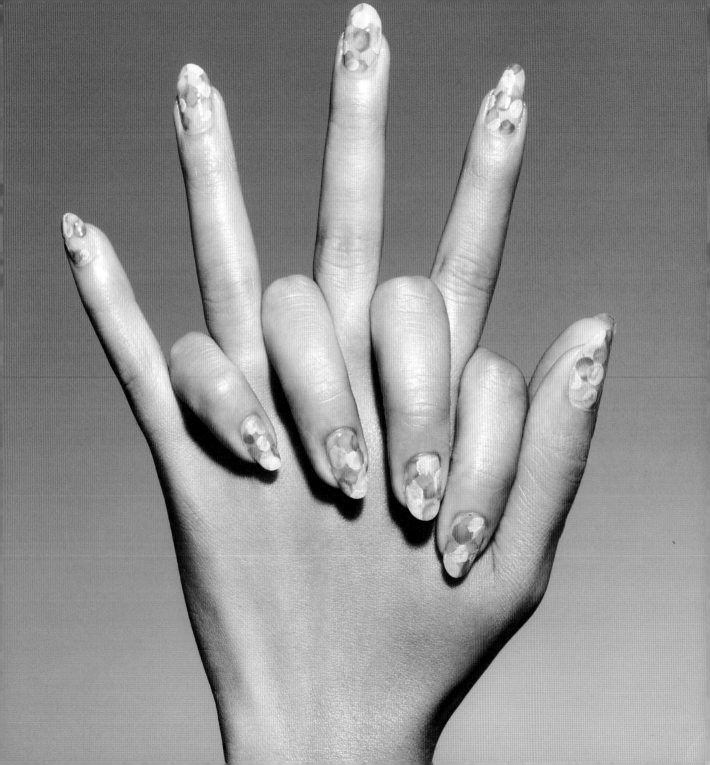

TRIANGULAR FUNK

The perfect party manicure features colorful triangles floating across the nails like confetti.

Tools

- Base coat
- Fine art brush
- Opaque white polish or acrylic paint
- Turquoise polish
- Light purple polish
- Top coat

1. Use a fine art brush to paint tiny triangles with opaque white polish. Place them across the entire nail, leaving lots of space in between. Let dry for two minutes.

2. Repeat Step 1 with turquoise polish, still leaving a bit of space in between the triangles. Let dry for two minutes.

3. Repeat Step 1 with light purple polish, filling in the spaces. Let dry for two minutes, then seal the design with top coat.

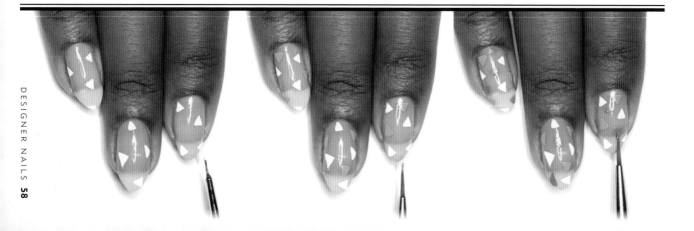

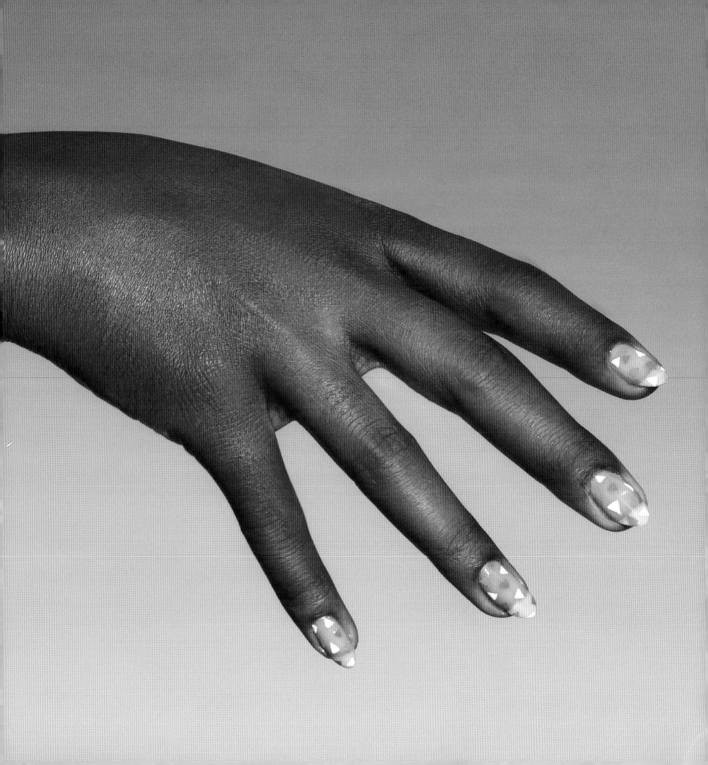

RACING STRIPES

Make fast tracks with this fun design that has lots of flair.

1. Working from base to tip, paint three squiggly lines diagonally across the nail with bright yellow polish. Let dry for two minutes.

2. With a fine art brush and black polish, paint thin squiggly line on top of the yellow, then outline the yellow stripes as well. The black lines should be randomly placed and abstract. Let dry for two minutes, then seal the design with top coat.

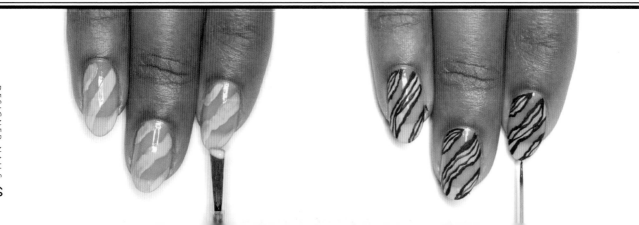

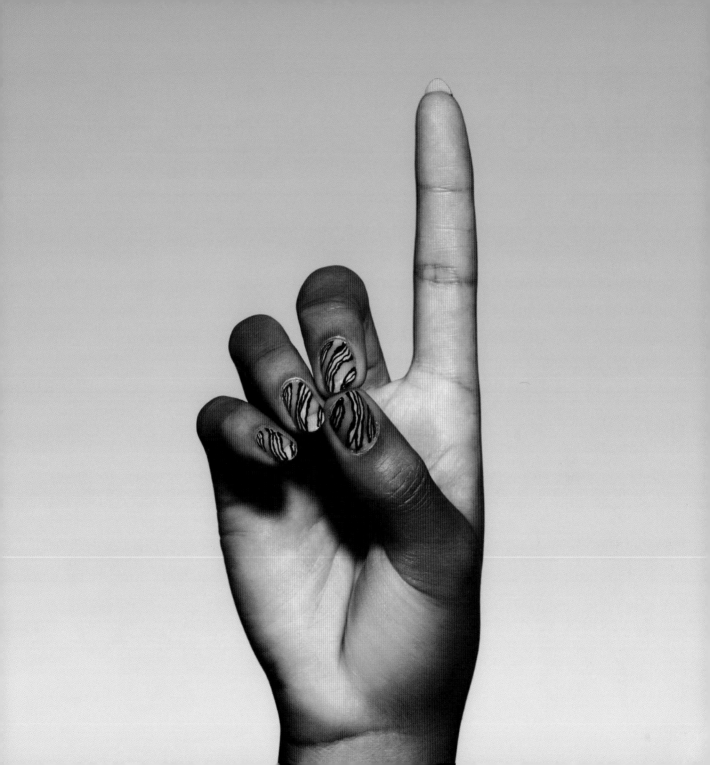

BLUE MOON

The white crescent at the base of the nail is called the *lunula*—it's Latin for "little moon." This design was painted with black and white polishes for the cover of this book. Here, blue moons and matching tips make an equally bold statement.

Tools

- Base coat
- Sheer nude polish
- Fine art brush
- Electric blue polish
- Top coat

1. Choose a sheer nude polish and apply two coats. Let dry for two minutes.

2. With a fine art brush and electric blue polish, trace the outline of the cuticle, then trace the half moon, outlining the shape of the natural moon. Fill in the outlined shape.

3. To create the French tip, use a fine art brush to outline the base of the nail tip, then fill it in to the top edge. Let dry for two minutes, then seal the design with top coat.

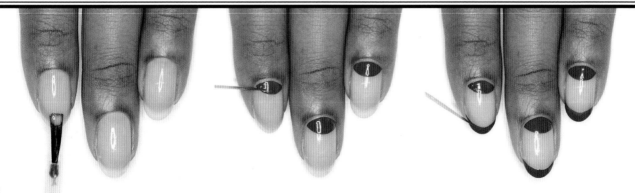

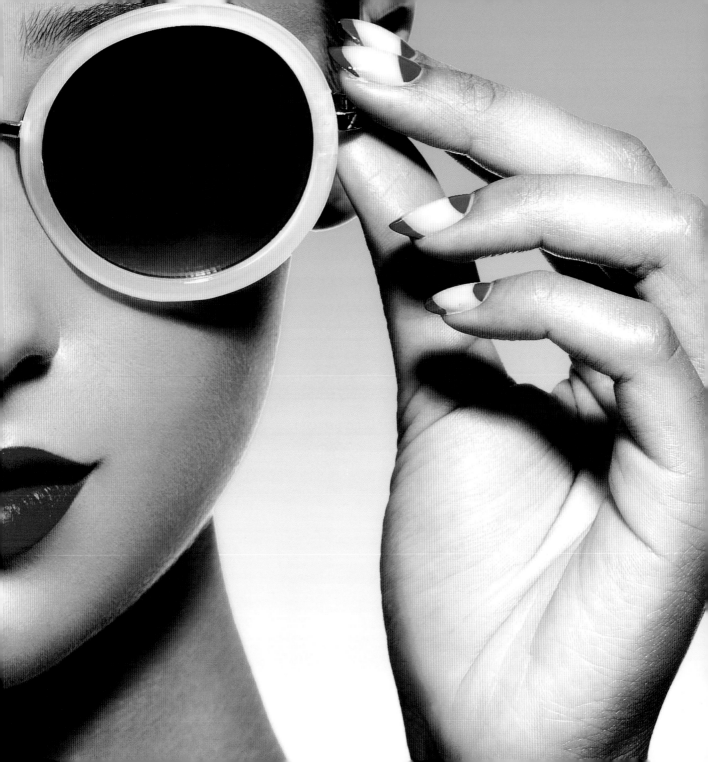

SPRING SPATTER

This design is pretty any time of year, but the pastel colors make me think of spring. To create this effect, it's important to control the amount of polish on the brush—less is more.

Tools

- ⌐ **Base coat**
- ⌐ **Lime green polish**
- ⌐ **Medium green polish**
- ⌐ **Opaque pink polish**
- ⌐ **Dark red polish**
- ⌐ **Top coat**

1. Apply two coats of lime green polish and let dry for two minutes.

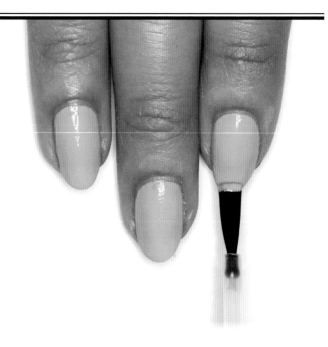

2. Wipe most of the medium green polish off its brush, then brush on random light strokes. Be sure to leave space for the colors that follow.

3. Repeat Step 2 with opaque pink polish. Again, wipe most of the polish off the brush, but overlap a bit onto the green strokes.

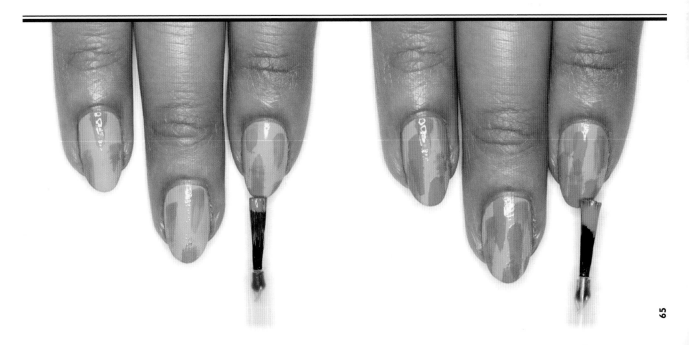

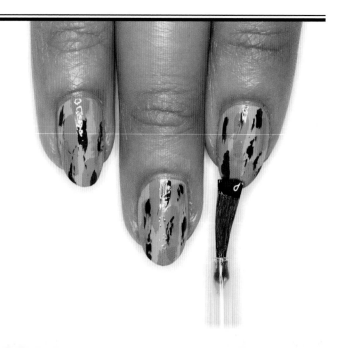

4. Repeat Step 2 with dark red polish, using very light, sparse strokes with almost no polish on the brush. Let dry for two minutes, then seal the design with top coat.

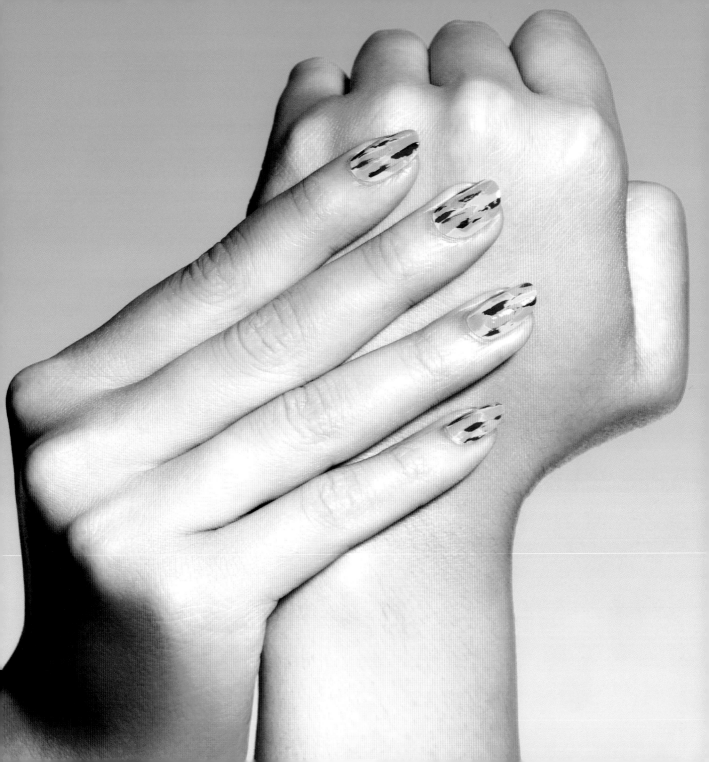

MODERN LINES

Think of this design as contemporary jewelry for your nails—a modern mix of metallic and bold colors.

Tools

- ⌐ **Base coat**
- ⌐ **Metallic copper polish**
- ⌐ **Opaque light blue polish**
- ⌐ **Fine art brush**
- ⌐ **Black polish or acrylic paint**
- ⌐ **Top coat**

1. Apply two coats of metallic copper polish and let dry for two minutes.

2. Paint two parallel lines of opaque light blue polish horizontally across the nail. Keep minimal polish on the brush to create even lines or use a fine art brush and fill in as you go.

3. With a fine art brush, outline the tops and bottoms of the blue bands with a line of black polish. Let dry for two minutes, then seal the design with top coat.

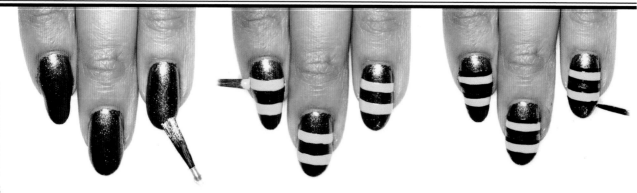

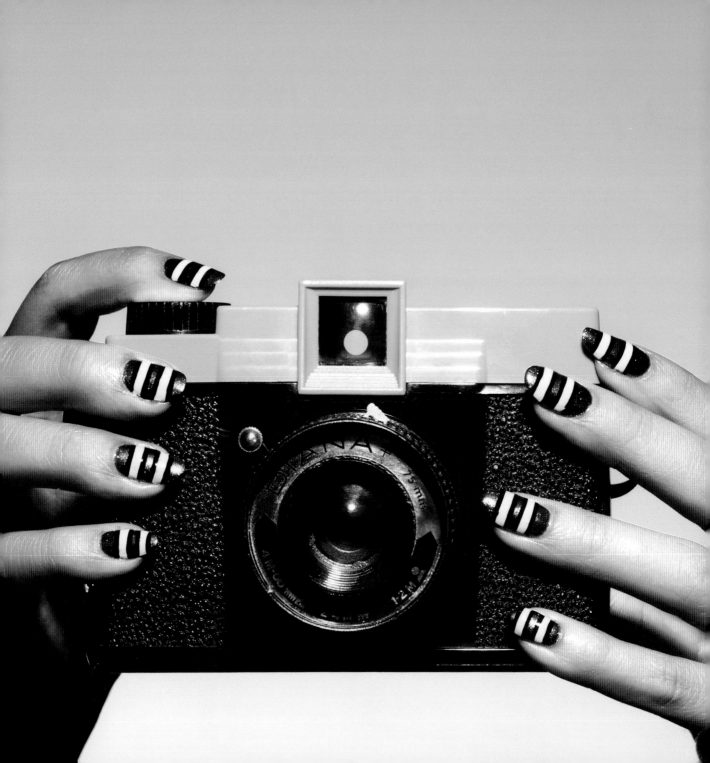

MONOCHROME FLOWERS

The tone-on-tone effect—achieved by painting gray flowers on a white background—looks like fine lace, while a dark blue French tip adds drama.

Tools

- ⌐ **Base coat**
- ⌐ **Opaque white polish**
- ⌐ **Fine art brush**
- ⌐ **Pale gray polish**
- ⌐ **Dark blue polish**
- ⌐ **Top coat**

1. Apply two coats of opaque white polish and let dry for two minutes.

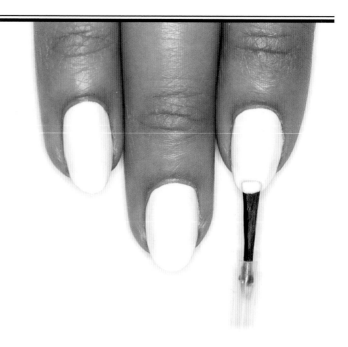

2. With a fine art brush and pale gray polish, paint abstract flowers. Start each flower by painting the center as a small circle, then surround the circle with abstract petal shapes. Feel free to vary the type of flower you paint.

3. Go back over any open spaces in your flowers, adding line patterns to fill in the space. Just take care not to fill them in completely. Let dry for two minutes.

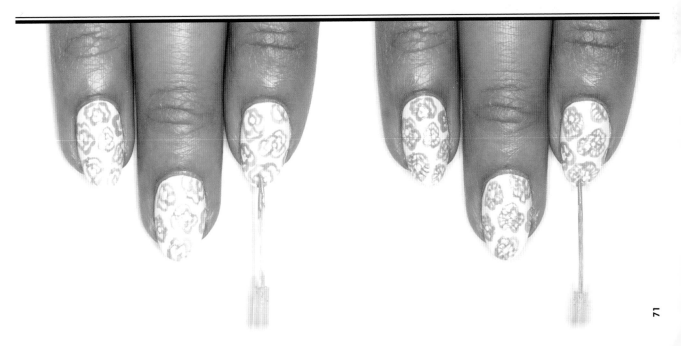

4. Paint the tip of the nail with dark blue polish to create a bold French tip. Let dry for two minutes, then seal the design with top coat.

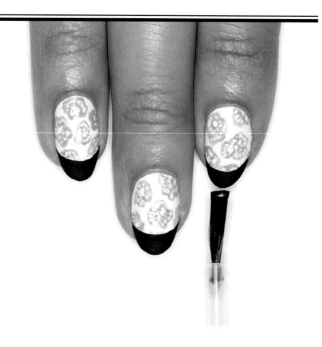

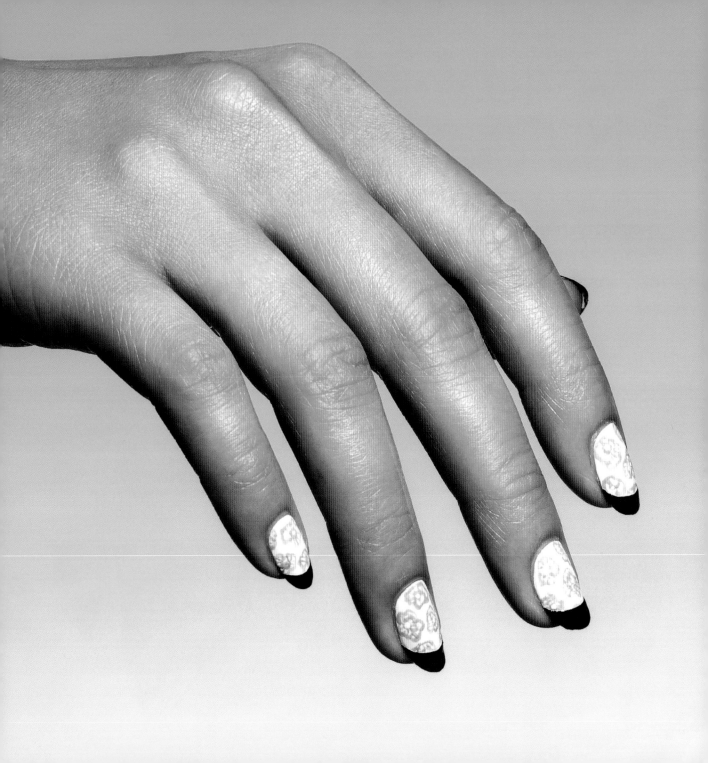

VIVID NUDE

Opaque nude polishes form a great base for bold shapes and striking contrasting colors like these.

Tools

- ¬ **Base coat**
- ¬ **Opaque nude polish**
- ¬ **Fine art brush**
- ¬ **Opaque yellow polish**
- ¬ **Opaque black polish or acrylic paint**
- ¬ **Top coat**

1. Apply two coats of opaque nude polish and let dry for two minutes.

2. With a fine art brush and opaque yellow polish, paint a line across the base of the nail (just above the top of the moon). Fill in the area from the line to the cuticle. Let dry for one minute.

3. With a fine art brush, paint a diagonal line of opaque black polish from one end of the yellow polish to the tip of the nail. Fill in the space completely, leaving only the top nude section exposed. Let dry for two minutes, then seal the design with top coat.

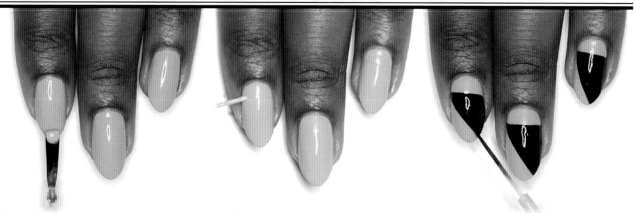

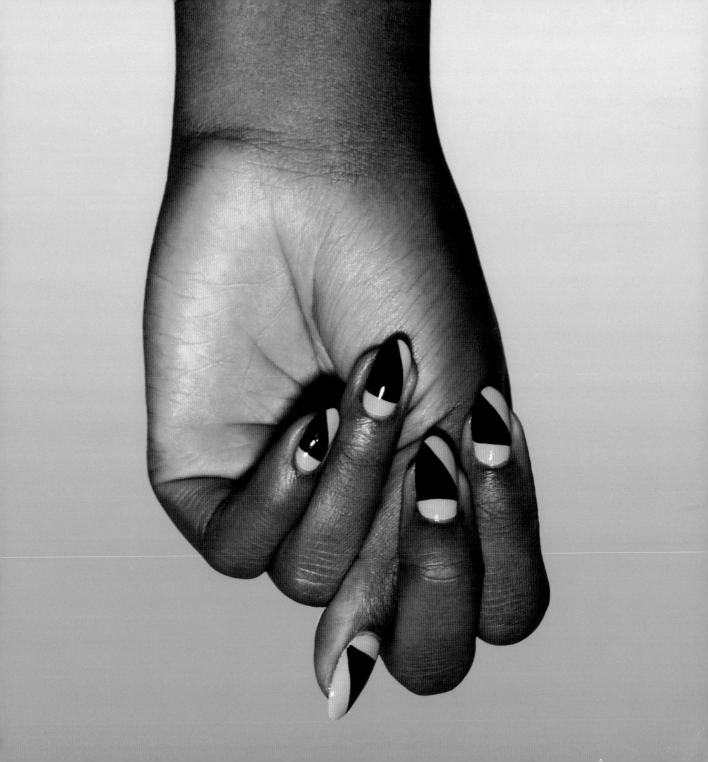

PÊCHE ET NOIR

This is a simple design with a lot of impact. The combination of peach and black is dramatic, but they're actually very neutral colors. I love the added effect of using both glossy and matte top coats.

Tools

- Base coat
- Opaque peach polish
- Fine art brush
- Black polish or acrylic paint
- Glossy top coat
- Matte-finish top coat

1. Apply two coats of opaque peach polish and let dry for two minutes.

2. With a fine art brush, paint a line of black polish down the center of the nail, then fill in one half of the nail with black polish. Let dry for two minutes; then, to take the look further, apply glossy top coat on the black half and matte-finish top coat on the peach half.

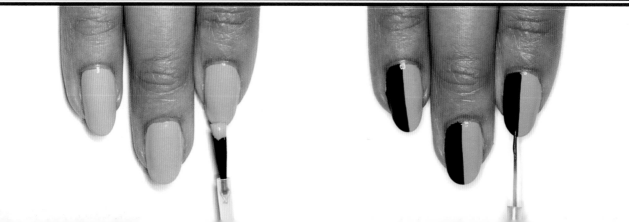

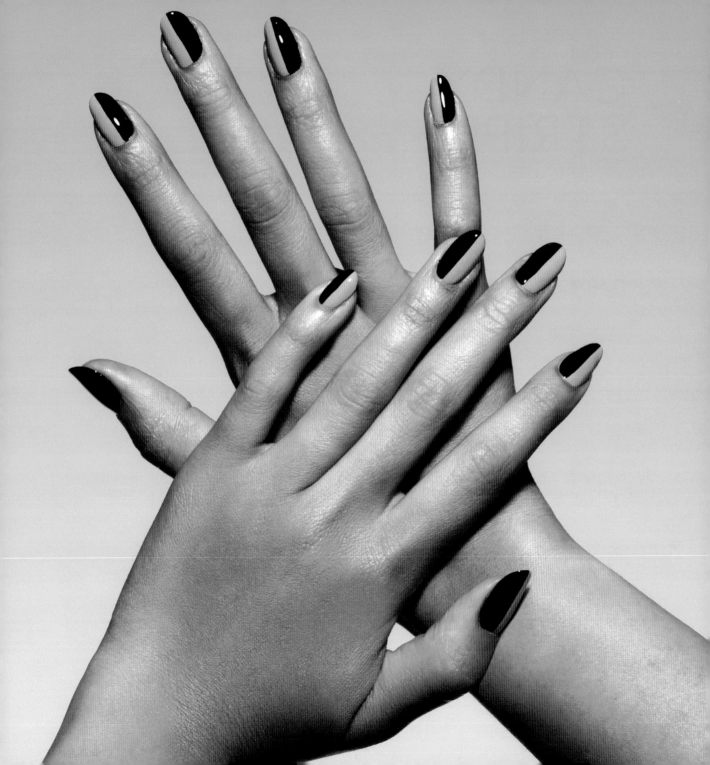

CANDY STRIPER

People will think you've dipped your hands in a bag of pink peppermint candy when you sport this fresh, delicious design.

1. With a fine art brush and bright red polish, paint vertical stripes of varying thickness. The center line should be thick, and the outside lines should be thin. Let dry for one minute.

2. With a fine art brush, paint a thick line of opaque bright pink polish on one side of the center red line, and a thin line parallel to one of the outer red lines. Let dry for one minute.

3. With a nail art brush and darker red polish, paint a thin line in the gap between the center line and the thin pink line. Let dry for two minutes, then seal the design with top coat.

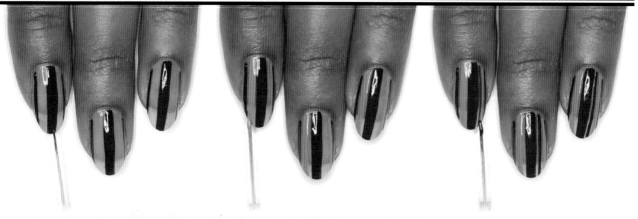

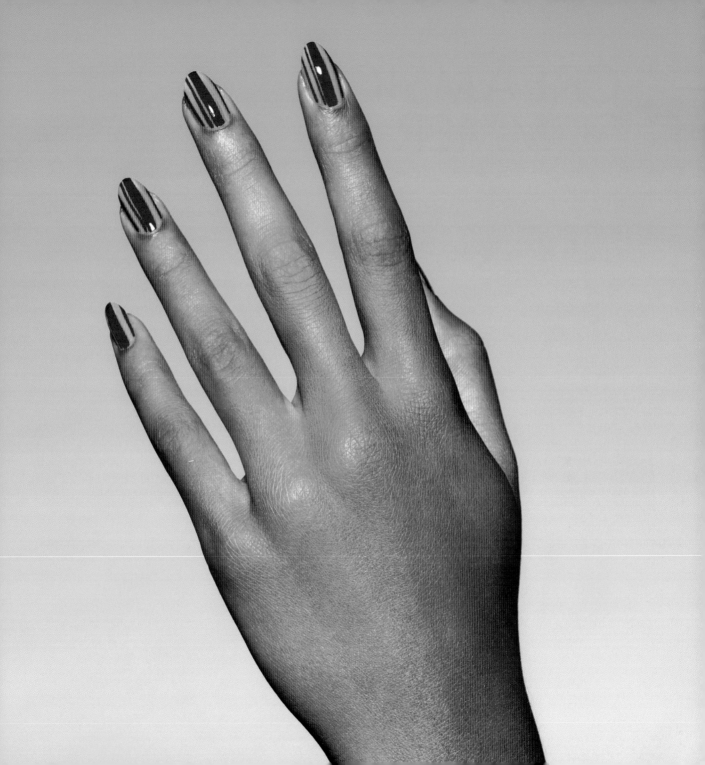

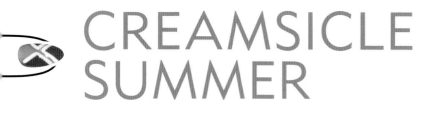

CREAMSICLE SUMMER

A refreshing design that's perfect for a summer day or a tropical vacation.

Tools

- ⌐ **Base coat**
- ⌐ **Fine art brush**
- ⌐ **Neon orange polish**
- ⌐ **Opaque white polish or acrylic paint**
- ⌐ **Top coat**

1. With a fine art brush and neon orange polish, paint three triangles. Paint one at the tip of the nail and then one on either side. Leave some space between them. Let dry for two minutes.

2. With a fine art brush, outline each triangle with a fairly thick line of opaque white polish. Let dry for two minutes, then seal the design with top coat.

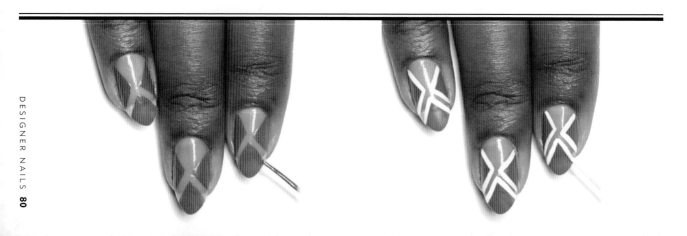

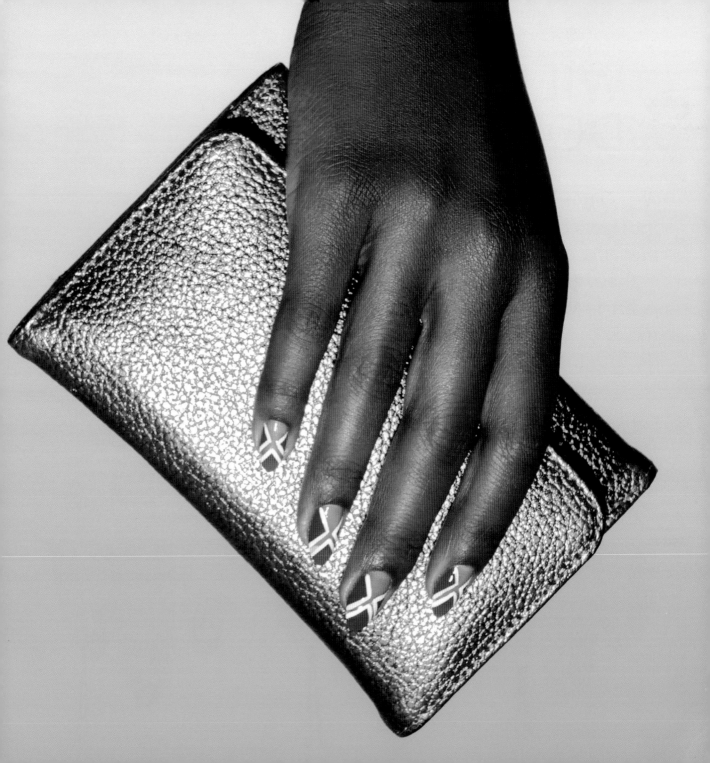

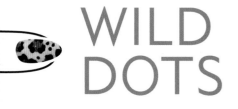

WILD DOTS

An easy-to-create animal print that gets extra shine from metallic copper polish. Choose a sheer nude for the best effect. A large bobby pin or a toothpick make great substitutes for the dotting tool.

Tools

- ⌐ **Base coat**
- ⌐ **Sheer nude polish**
- ⌐ **Dotting tool**
- ⌐ **Metallic copper polish**
- ⌐ **Black polish or acrylic paint**
- ⌐ **Top coat**

1. Apply two coats of sheer nude polish. Let dry for two minutes.

2. With the larger end of the dotting tool and metallic copper polish, create a pattern of random dots across the nail. Be sure to leave some space between the dots.

3. With the smaller end of the dotting tool, trace the metallic copper dots with dots of black polish to create a cheetah print. Paint random small dots in between the larger spots as well. Let dry for two minutes, then seal the design with top coat.

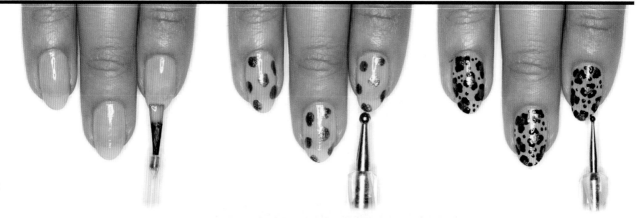

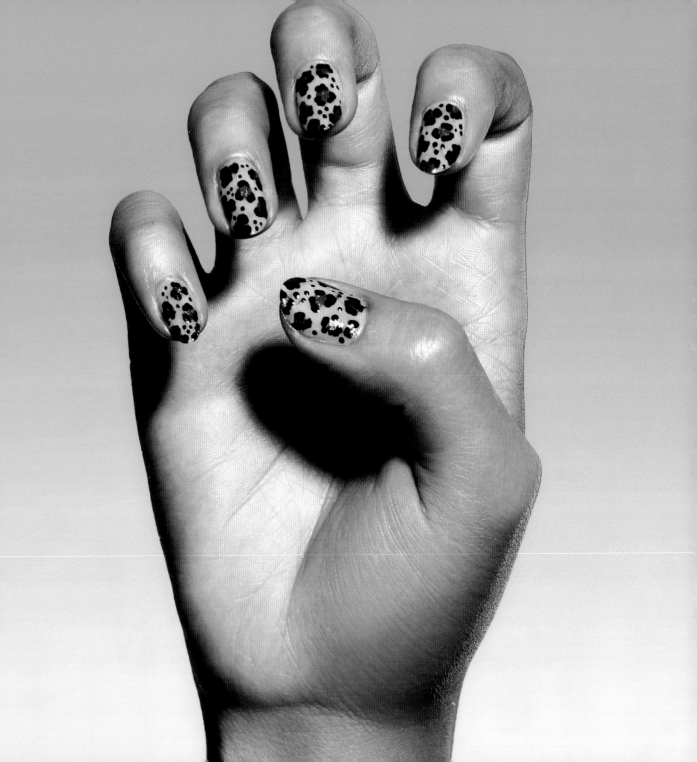

24K FLOWERS

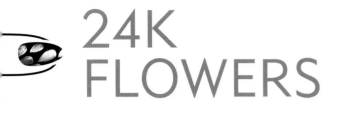

Like flower petals floating on the wind, these sparkling teardrop shapes bring a sense of movement to your fingertips.

Tools

- ¬ **Base coat**
- ¬ **Metallic dark blue polish**
- ¬ **Fine art brush**
- ¬ **Metallic pale gold polish**
- ¬ **Top coat**

2. Working from the base of the nail toward the tip, use a fine art brush and metallic pale gold polish to paint teardrop shapes. To create the teardrop shape, paint a triangle first, then round out the bottom by painting a half circle at the base of the triangle. Leave one side of the tip exposed to give the design a sense of motion. Let dry for two minutes, then seal the design with top coat.

1. Apply two coats of metallic dark blue polish and let dry for two minutes.

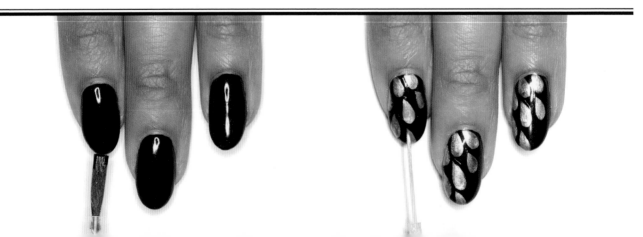

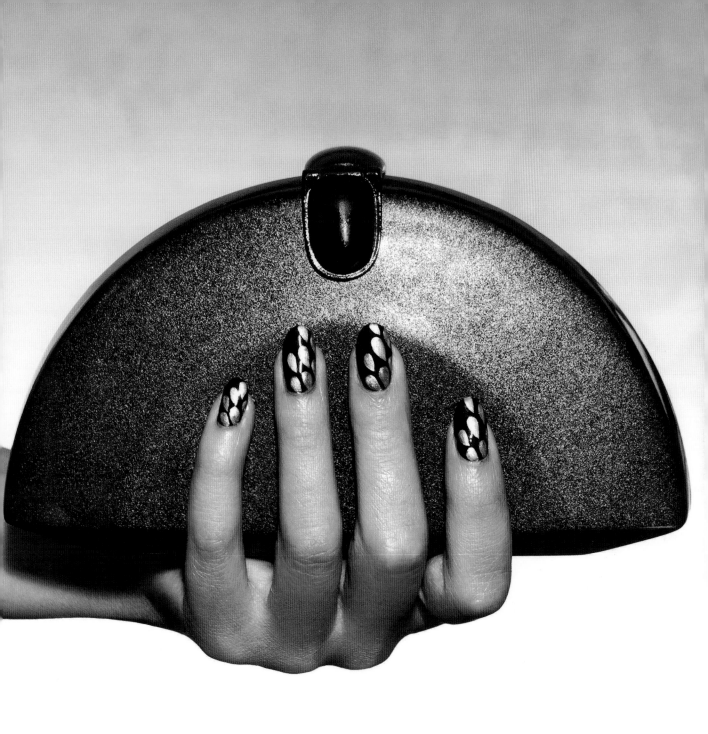

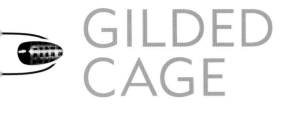

GILDED CAGE

Black and metallic are a great combination, and this design is dressy enough for nights out but simple enough for every day.

Tools

- Base coat
- Black polish or acrylic paint
- Fine art brush
- Metallic gold polish
- Top coat

1. Apply two coats of black polish and let dry for two minutes.

2. With a fine art brush and metallic gold polish, paint a rectangle shape with its bottom edge a little closer to the cuticle than the center of the nail; leave it open at the tip.

3. Paint a grid pattern of vertical and horizontal lines inside the rectangle. Let dry for two minutes, then seal the design with top coat.

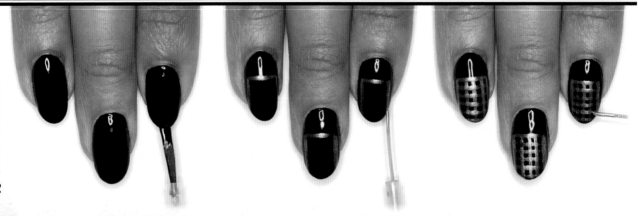

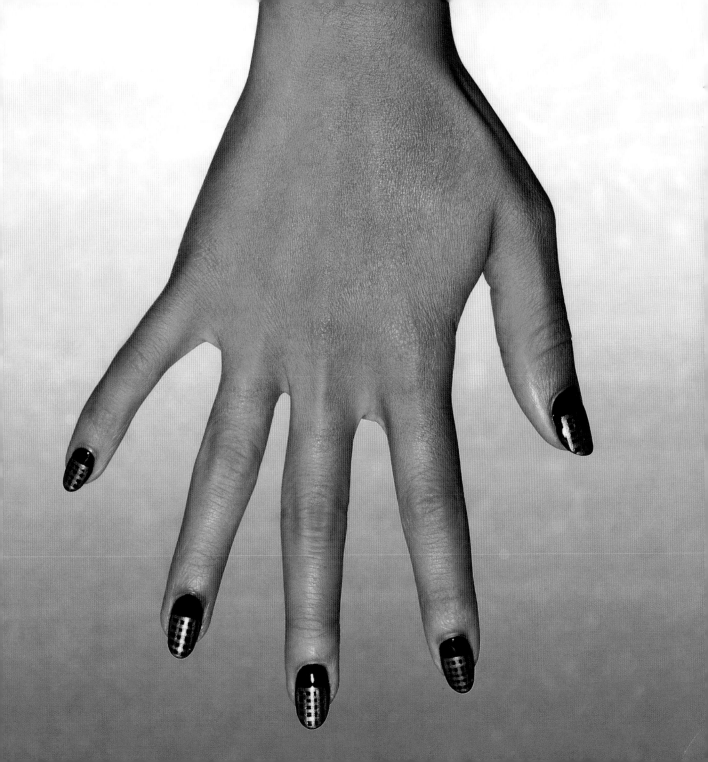

MATTE CHIC

This design plays with shiny and matte finishes. The matte-finish top coat adds richness to the black, which is offset by pale gold, glittery tips.

Tools

- ⌐ **Base coat**
- ⌐ **Fine art brush**
- ⌐ **Opaque black polish**
- ⌐ **Matte-finish top coat**
- ⌐ **Pale metallic gold polish with fine glitter**
- ⌐ **Top coat**

1. With a fine art brush and opaque black polish, outline the top of the moon, then paint the nail to the tip, leaving the half moon exposed. Let dry for two minutes.

2. Apply one coat of matte-finish top coat and let dry for three minutes.

3. Using a fine art brush and pale metallic gold polish with fine glitter, paint a French tip at the top of your nail. Let dry for two minutes, then paint the gold tip with regular top coat to give it contrast and shine.

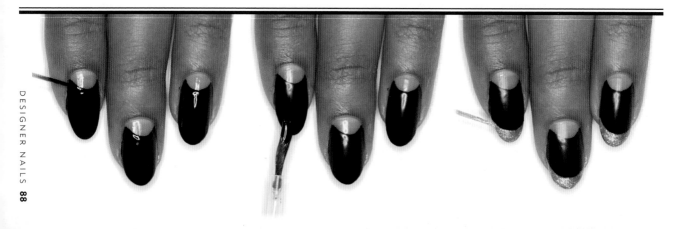

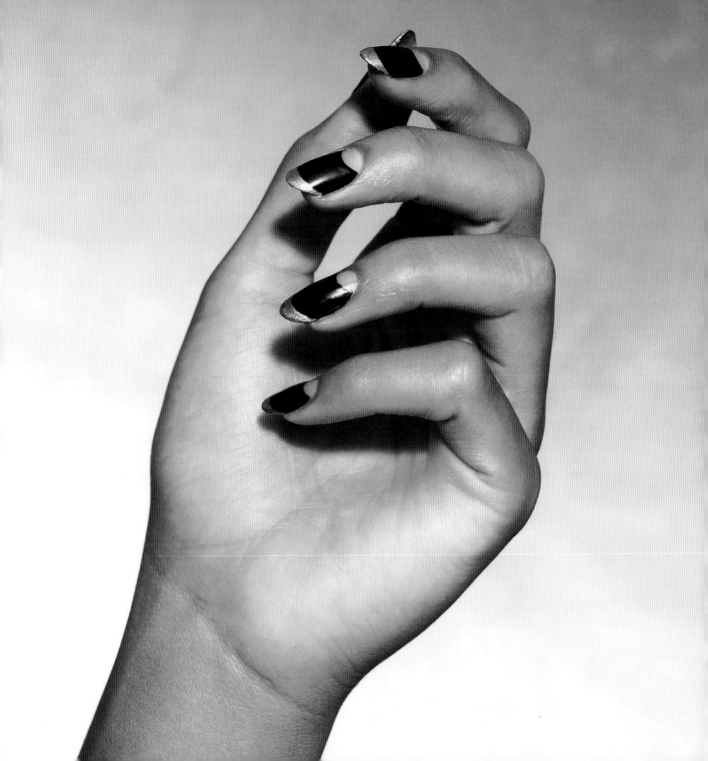

COLOR GRID

Rich colors become even more luxe with an outline of metallic gold—the result is a fashionable coat of arms.

Tools

- ¬ **Base coat**
- ¬ **Opaque peach polish**
- ¬ **Fine art brush**
- ¬ **Dark blue polish**
- ¬ **Dark red polish**
- ¬ **Dark green polish**
- ¬ **Metallic gold polish**
- ¬ **Top coat**

1. Apply two coats of opaque peach polish and let dry for two minutes.

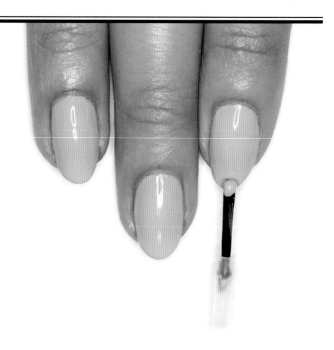

2. Wipe most of the dark blue polish off its brush, then paint a dark blue box on the bottom quarter of the nail. Use the fine art brush for this if you find it easier. Let dry for two minutes.

3. Working as in Step 2 and leaving a line space between the colors, paint a dark red box on the other bottom quarter of the nail and then a dark green box on the top quarter. The fourth quarter remains peach.

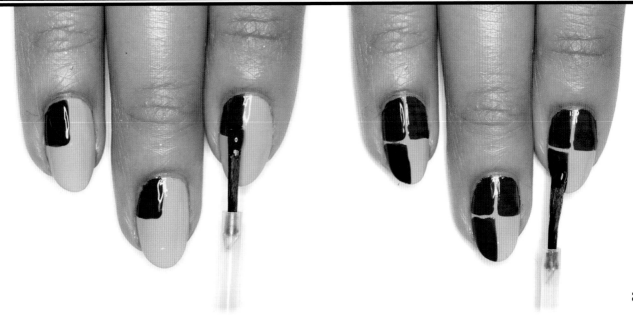

4. With a fine art brush and metallic gold polish, paint lines to fill the gaps between all four colors. Let dry for two minutes, then seal the design with top coat.

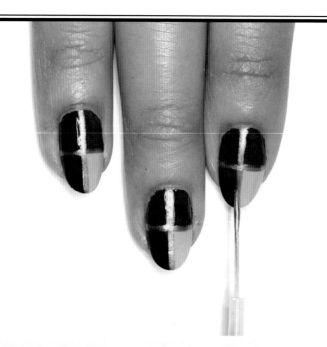

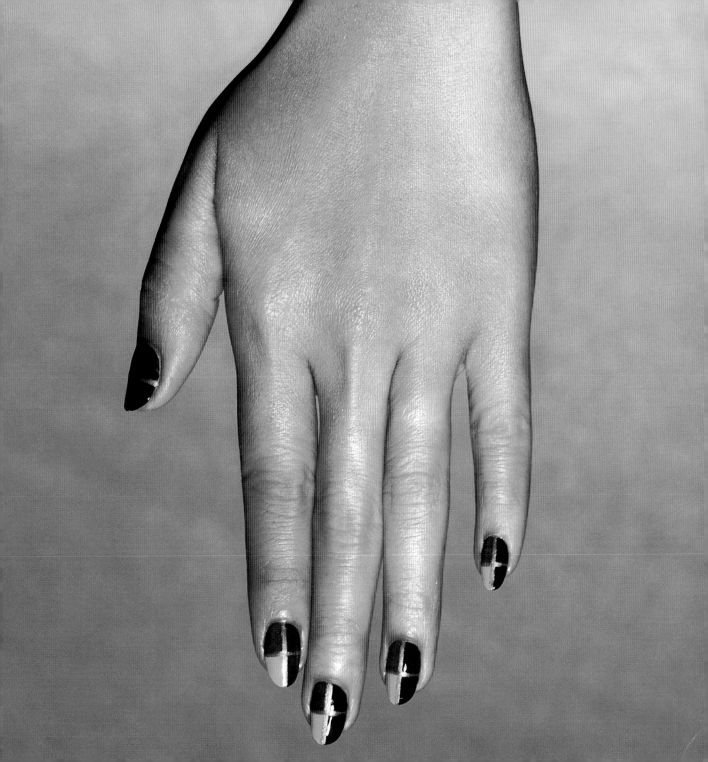

GOLD FINGER

These nails are glamorous enough for any Bond girl, thanks to three different shades of gold polish. Using polishes with small- and large-size glitter adds an extra dimension of shine.

Tools

⌐ **Base coat**

⌐ **Deep gold metallic polish**

⌐ **Pale gold polish with chunky glitter**

⌐ **Bright gold polish with fine glitter**

⌐ **Fine art brush**

⌐ **Opaque white polish or acrylic paint**

⌐ **Top coat**

1. Apply two coats of deep gold metallic polish and let dry for two minutes.

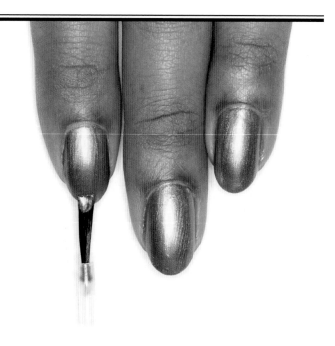

2. Using pale gold polish with chunky glitter, brush up one side of the nail from the cuticle. Stop halfway between the cuticle and the tip.

3. Using bright gold polish with fine glitter, paint around the pale gold, working almost in a J shape. Note that only two thirds of the base color is covered. Let dry for one minute.

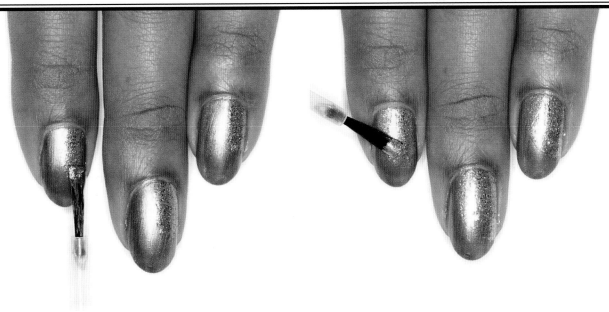

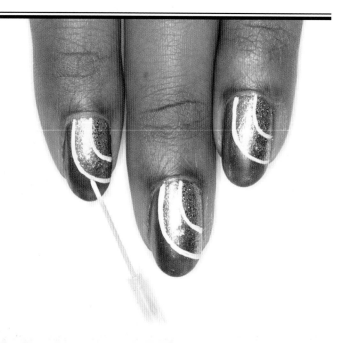

4. With a fine art brush and opaque white polish, outline the first and second colors, repeating the J formation. Let dry for two minutes, then seal the design with top coat.

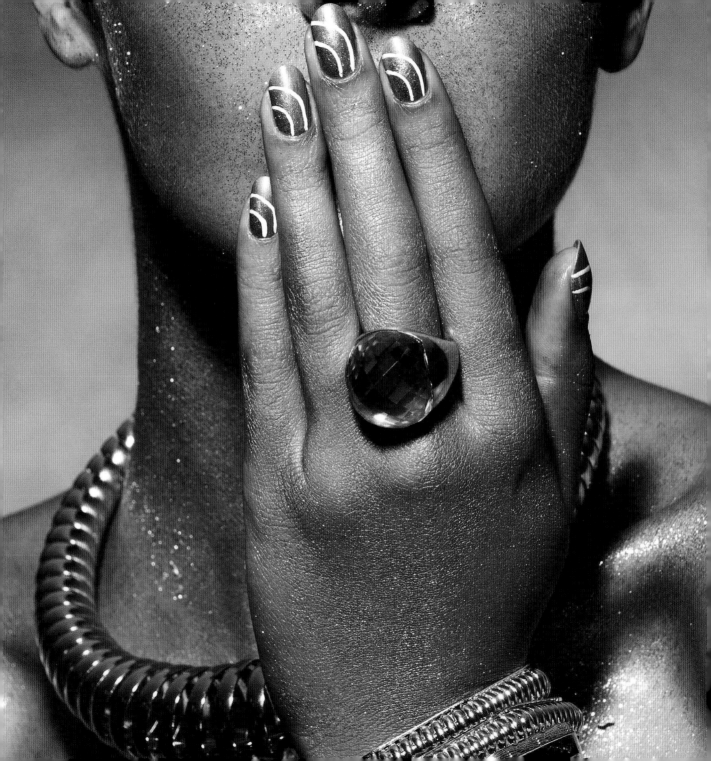

LEAFY GREENS

Go back to nature with a shimmery twist. With its dark background, this pattern is reminiscent of a vintage fabric design.

Tools

- ⌐ **Base coat**
- ⌐ **Dark shimmery green polish**
- ⌐ **Opaque pale green polish**
- ⌐ **Fine art brush**
- ⌐ **Top coat**

1. Apply two coats of dark shimmery green polish and let dry for two minutes.

2. With opaque pale green polish, paint random strokes over the entire nail. Leave some space between the shapes, but don't worry about being too neat.

3. With a fine art brush and dark shimmery green polish, define the leaf shapes, first by outlining the edges and then by adding veins to the leaves. Let dry for two minutes, then seal the design with top coat.

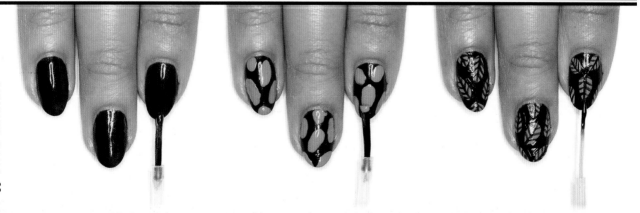

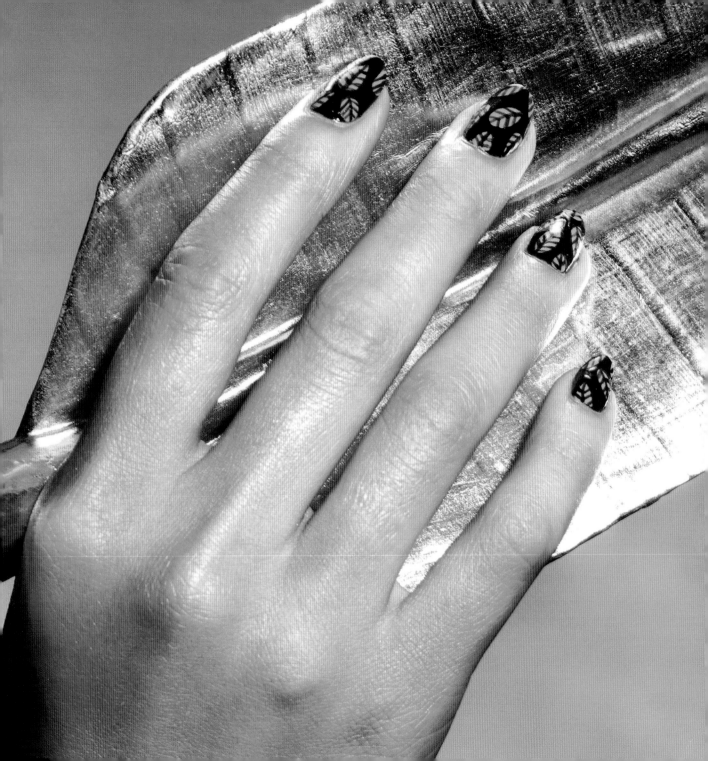

LUXE DOTS

This pretty design is so simple to create. It's a great starting point for the beginning nail artist. Use a toothpick if you don't have a dotting tool.

Tools

- Base coat
- Metallic gold polish with fine glitter
- Dotting tool or toothpick
- Black polish or acrylic paint
- Top coat

1. Apply two coats of metallic gold polish with fine glitter and let dry for two minutes.

2. With the smaller end of a dotting tool and black polish, create polka dots covering the entire nail. For the best alignment, start your first dot at the base of the nail and complete a straight row up to the tip, then paint the adjoining dots to the left and the right of that row. Let dry for two minutes, then seal the design with top coat.

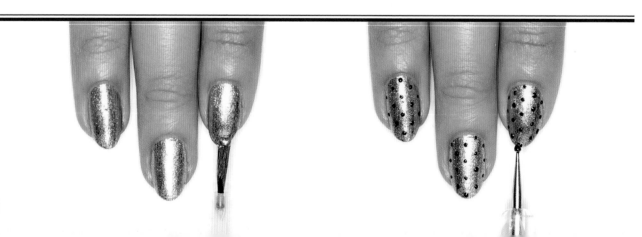

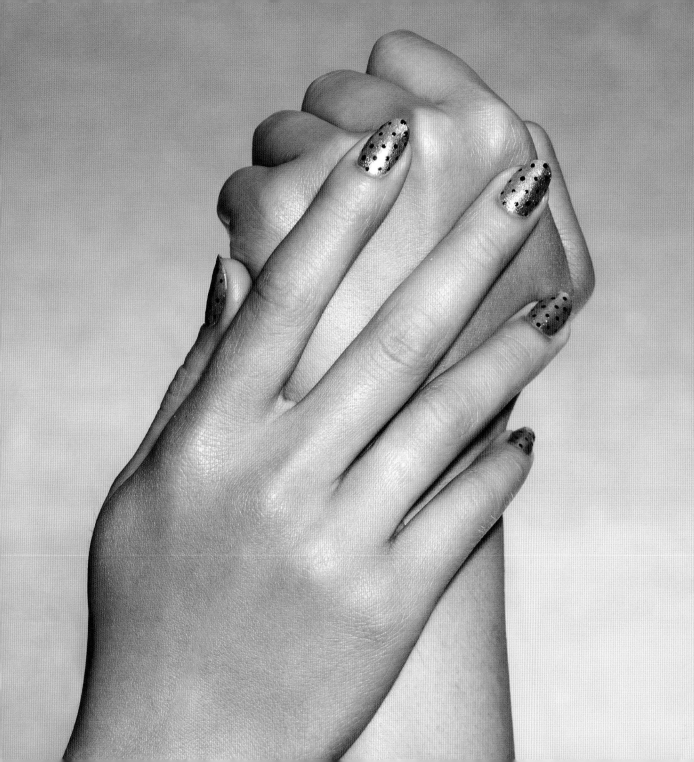

NEUTRAL CENTER

Subtle, pretty colors dotted with metallic make for a design with mysterious allure.

Tools

- ¬ **Base coat**
- ¬ **Sheer nude polish**
- ¬ **Taupe polish**
- ¬ **Brown polish**
- ¬ **Metallic gold polish with fine glitter**
- ¬ **Top coat**

1. Apply two coats of sheer nude polish and let dry for two minutes.

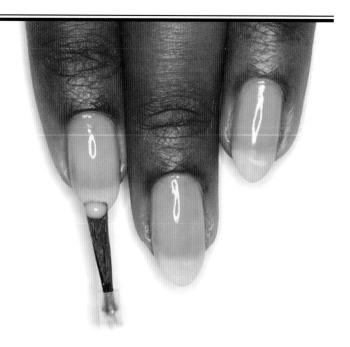

2. With taupe polish, paint an oval shape in the center of the nail. Keep the edges irregular; it does not have to be perfect. Let dry for one minute.

3. With brown polish, paint a smaller oval shape over the taupe polish. Let dry for one minute.

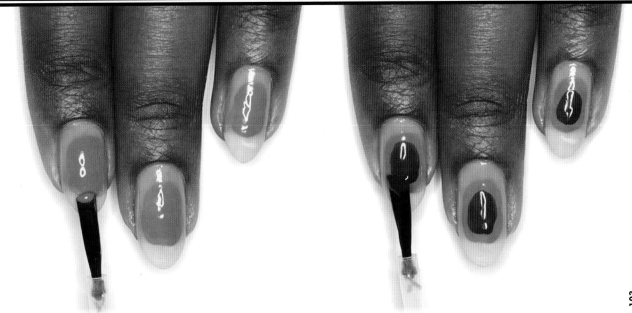

4. Using metallic gold polish with fine glitter, paint a smaller oval shape over the brown polish. Let dry for two minutes, then seal the design with top coat.

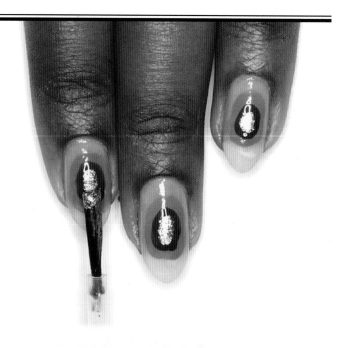

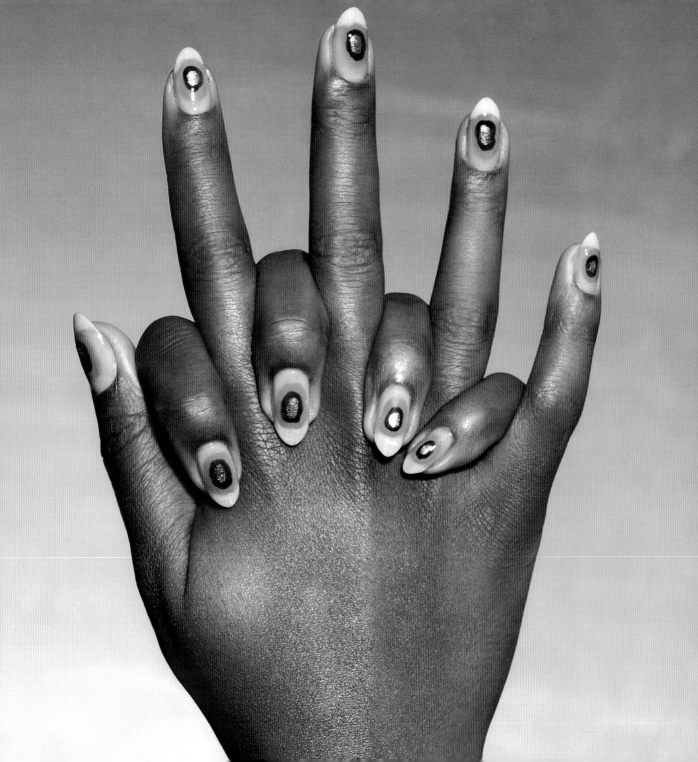

SPOT MADNESS

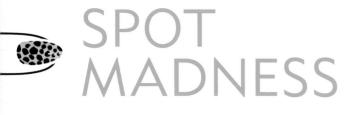

Make an animal print even wilder by painting the pattern over a pair of contrasting colors.

Tools

- ⌐ **Base coat**
- ⌐ **Opaque nude polish**
- ⌐ **Bright light blue polish**
- ⌐ **Thin fine art brush**
- ⌐ **Opaque black polish or acrylic paint**
- ⌐ **Top coat**

3. With a thin fine art brush and opaque black polish, paint small dots, varying the size and shape, across the entire nail. Let dry for two minutes, then seal the design with top coat.

1. Apply two coats of opaque nude polish and let dry for two minutes.

2. Paint one side of the nail with bright light blue polish and let dry for two minutes.

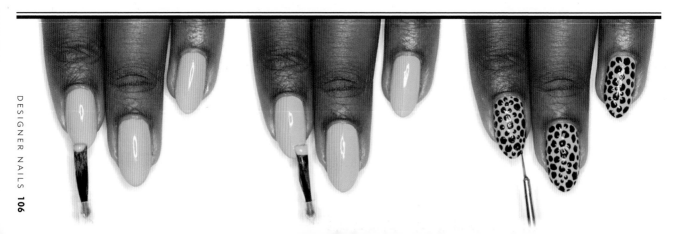

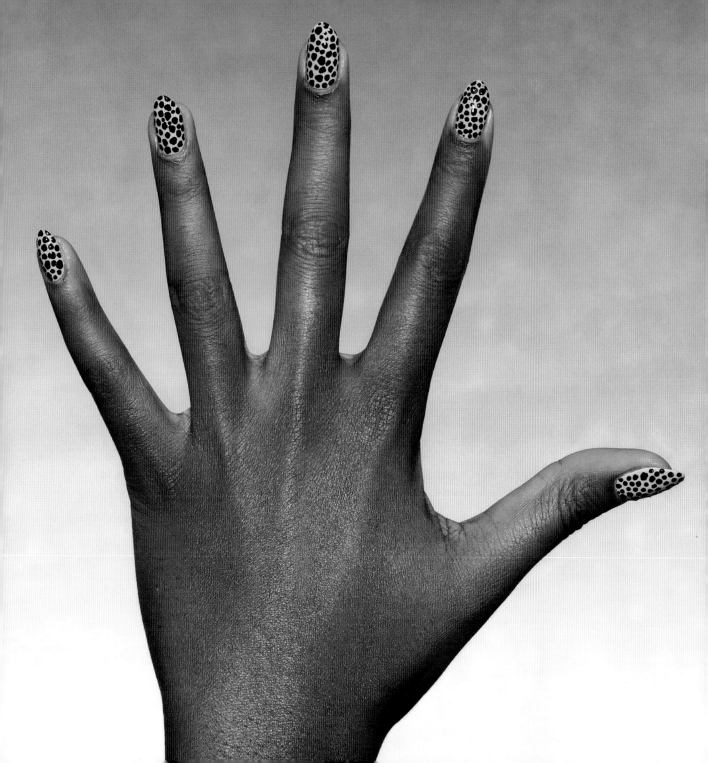

BDQ

This design is an homage to the jewelry featured in the photograph on the facing page, a custom-designed piece by Bande des Quatres. Gray and silver are an elegant combination, but experiment with other primary colors, too.

Tools

⌐ **Base coat**

⌐ **Metallic silver polish**

⌐ **Fine art brush**

⌐ **Dark gray polish**

⌐ **Top coat**

1. Apply two coats of metallic silver polish and let dry for two minutes.

2. With a fine art brush and dark gray polish, paint a honeycomb pattern all over the nail. Let dry for two minutes.

3. Paint two lines, from the center point to the sides, inside each honeycomb shape to create a triangle inside the shape. Let dry for two minutes, then seal the design with top coat.

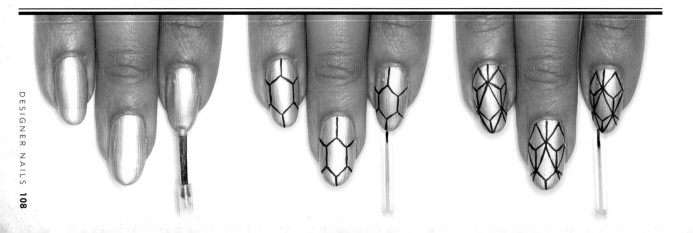

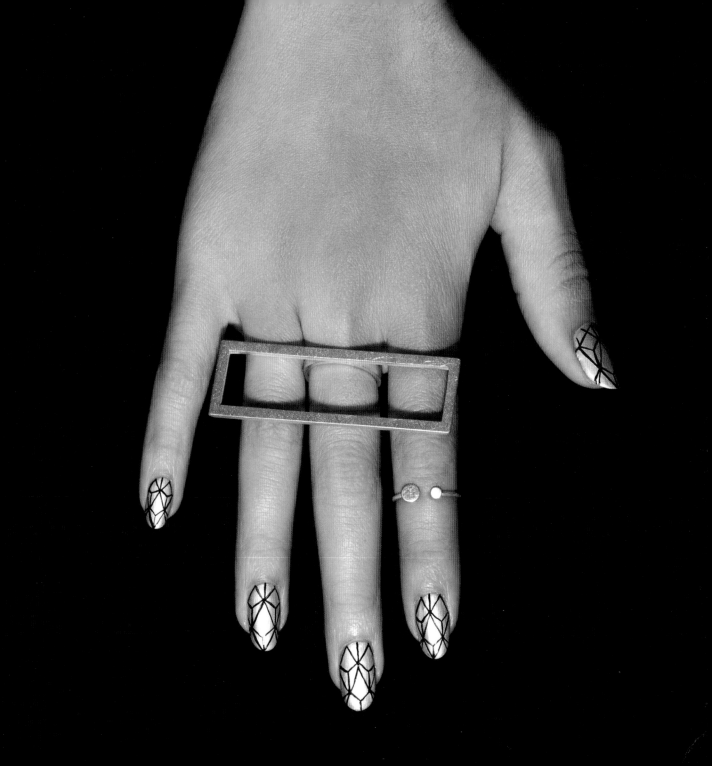

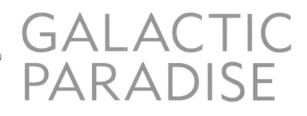

GALACTIC PARADISE

The universe is in your hands, as each nail sports its own private galaxy. This is a simple design that makes great use of iridescence and glitter.

Tools

- Opaque black polish or acrylic paint
- Iridescent green polish
- Sheer polish with fine silver glitter
- Sheer nude polish
- Very thin fine art brush
- Opaque white polish or acrylic paint
- Top coat

1. Apply two coats of opaque black polish and let dry for two minutes.

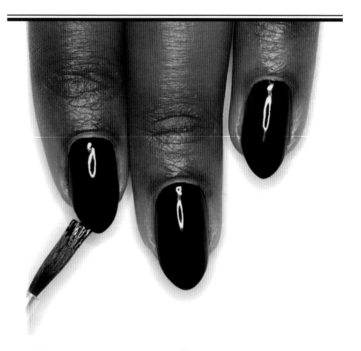

2. Paint a fat irregular line of iridescent green polish down the center of the nail by tapping the brush lightly as you move from the cuticle to the nail tip.

3. Paint each side of the nail with sheer polish with fine silver glitter, overlapping slightly on either side of the iridescent green.

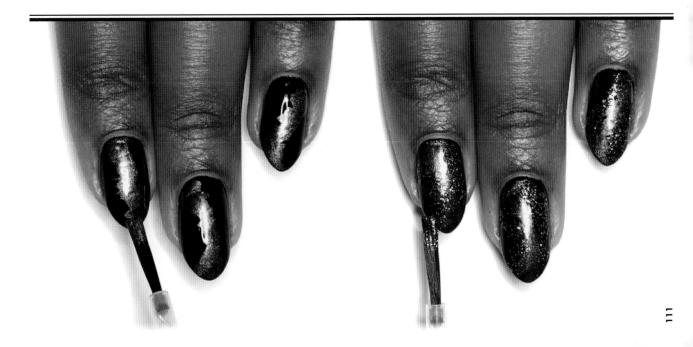

4. Use the polish brush to paint random large dots of sheer nude polish across the nail, leaving a good amount of space between the dots. You want these shapes to be irregular, so use the brush rather than a dotting tool.

5. Using a very thin fine art brush to achieve small specks, paint one tiny dot of opaque white polish inside each of the larger nude dots and then all across the nail to create the stars. Let dry for two minutes, then seal the design with top coat.

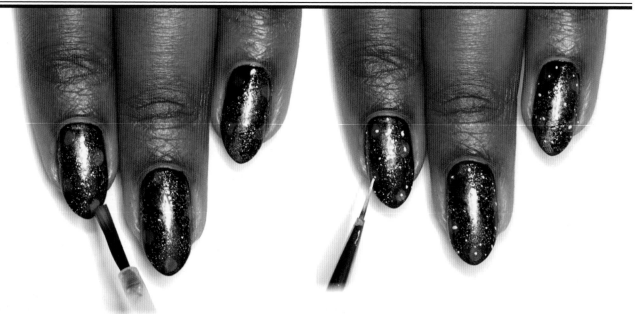

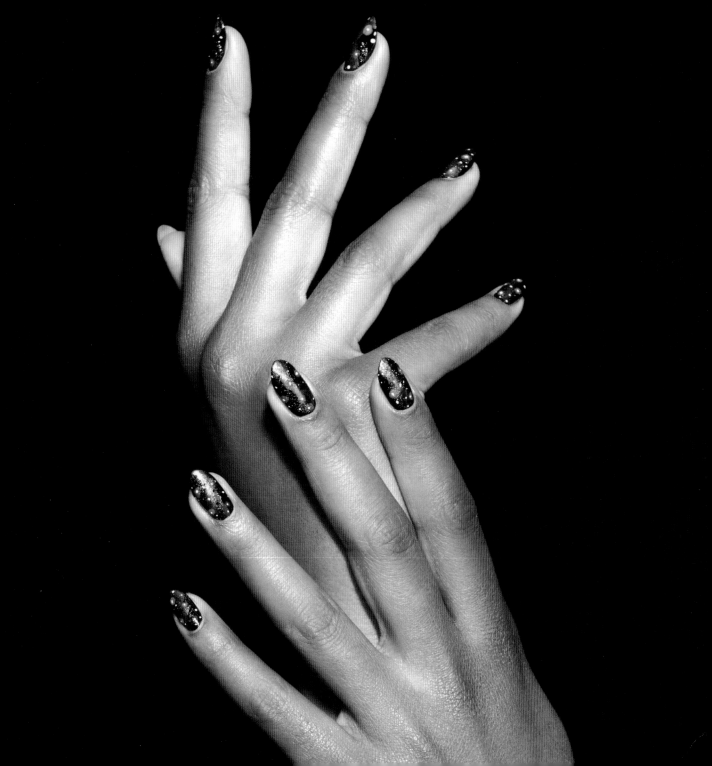

LUXE EXPOSED

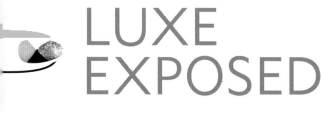

A fashionable take on a harlequin print; the gold tip adds a touch of glamour.

Tools

- ⌐ **Base coat**
- ⌐ **Fine art brush**
- ⌐ **Metallic gold polish with fine glitter**
- ⌐ **Opaque white polish or acrylic paint**
- ⌐ **Opaque black polish or acrylic paint**
- ⌐ **Top coat**

1. Using a fine art brush and metallic gold polish with fine glitter, paint a triangle shape at the very tip of the nail. Let dry for one minute.

2. With a fine art brush and opaque white polish, create another triangle to one side of the first triangle. Let dry for one minute.

3. Repeat Step 2 with opaque black polish opposite the white triangle. Let dry for two minutes, then seal the design with top coat.

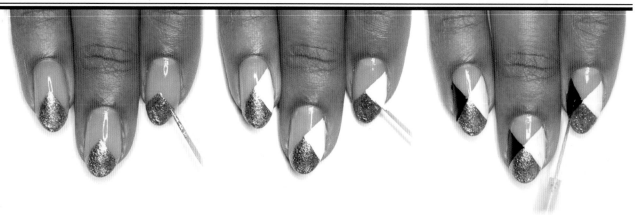

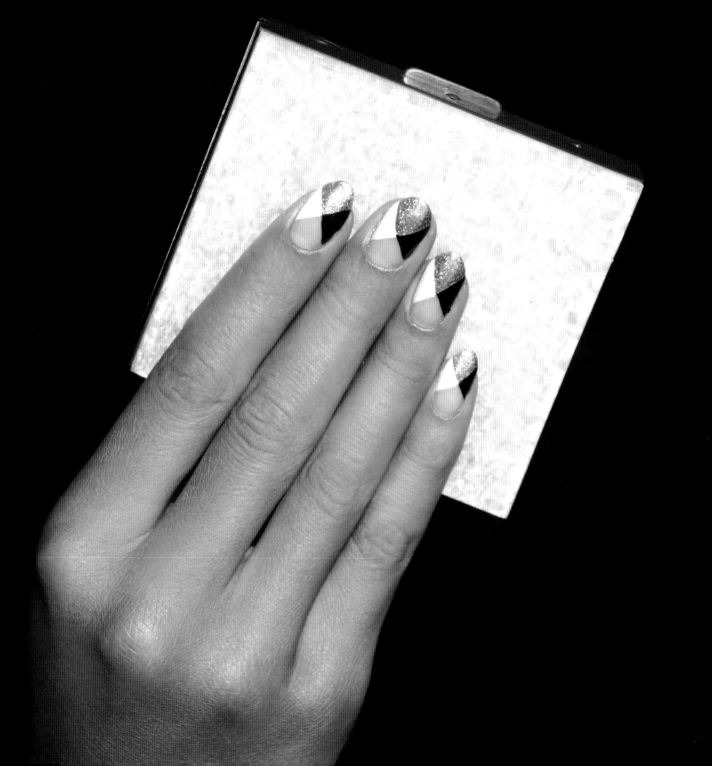

NEON
LIGHTS

Talk about vivid! Here's a simple design that will make the most of a night out—a French tip of neon polish that will glow in the dark.

Tools

- Base coat
- Pale nude polish
- Neon yellow polish
- Clear glow-in-the-dark top coat
- Top coat

2. Paint a French tip over your natural nail tip with one coat of neon yellow polish. Let dry for one minute. Paint the French tip with clear glow-in-the-dark top coat. Let dry for two minutes, then seal the design with regular top coat.

1. Apply two coats of pale nude polish and let dry for two minutes.

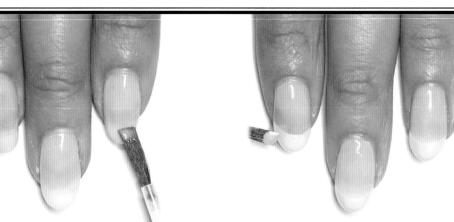

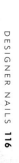

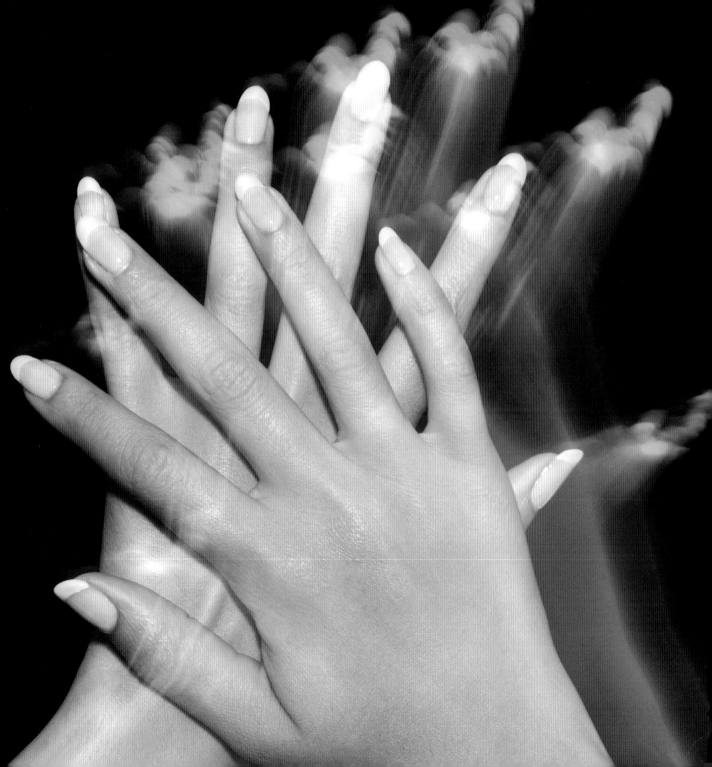

RAYS OF RED

Combine shades of peach, red, and coral to create a mini-sunburst on every nail.

Tools

- Base coat
- Opaque bright peach polish
- Fine art brush
- Red polish
- Coral polish
- Top coat

1. Using opaque bright peach polish, paint a stripe from the center edge of the nail to the tip, keeping the brush at an angle. Let dry for one minute.

2. With a fine art brush and red polish, paint a line next to the peach polish, making the line thinner as it moves to the top of the nail. Fill in the open space and let dry for one minute.

3. Repeat Step 2 with coral polish. Let dry for two minutes, then seal the design with top coat.

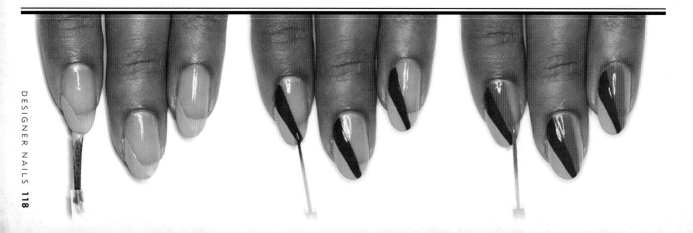

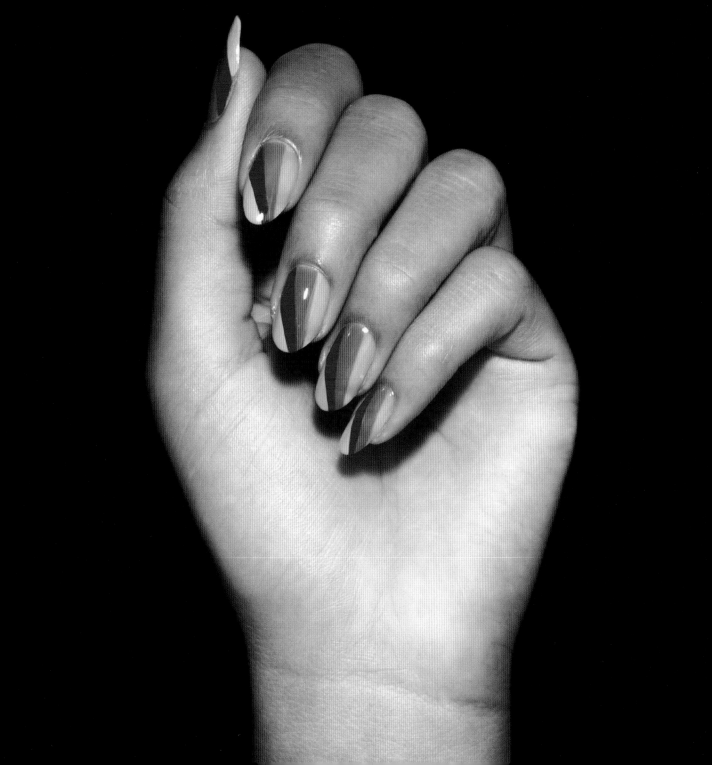

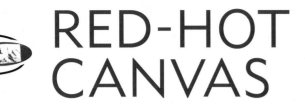

RED-HOT CANVAS

The beautiful abstract design lends itself to many color combinations—it's another example of the nail as canvas.

Tools

⌐ **Base coat**

⌐ **Opaque white polish or acrylic paint**

⌐ **Opaque black polish or acrylic paint**

⌐ **Fine art brush**

⌐ **Bright red polish**

⌐ **Top coat**

1. Apply two coats of opaque white polish and let dry for two minutes.

2. Wipe most of the opaque black polish off its brush, then dab the remainder across the center of the nail. Work randomly, but contain the black to a rectangular area.

3. With a fine art brush and bright red polish, paint a frame up the sides of the nail and across the tip. Let dry for two minutes, then seal the design with top coat.

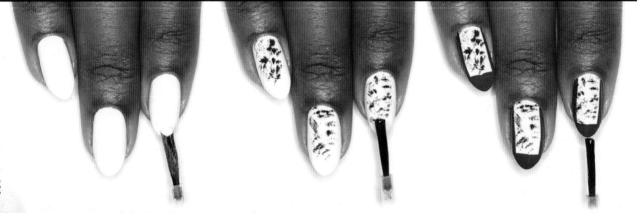

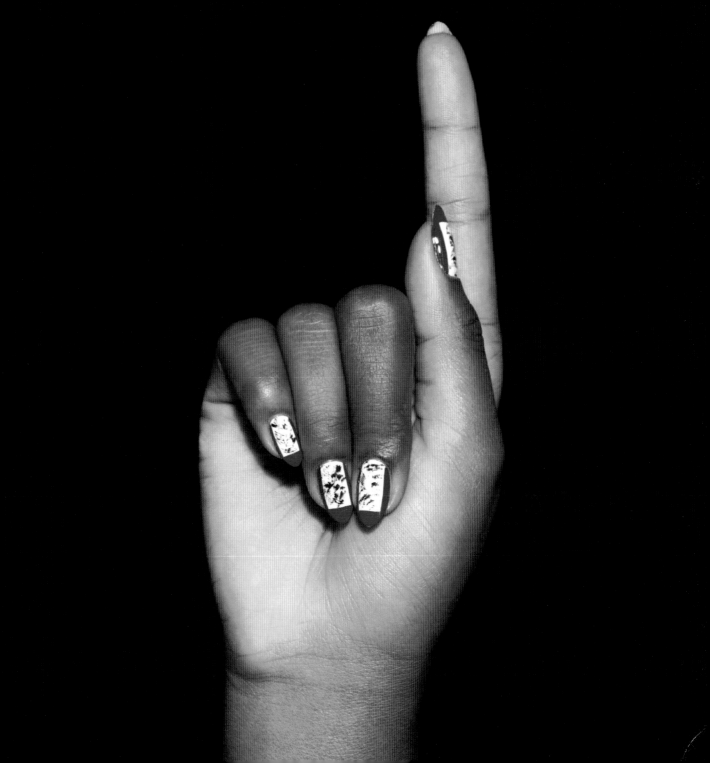

TUMBLING TILES

I love it when designs give a sense of movement. Here, it looks like the tiles of color are tumbling from the tips of the nails.

Tools

- ⌐ **Base coat**
- ⌐ **Dusty rose polish**
- ⌐ **Dark burgundy polish**
- ⌐ **Top coat**

1. Apply two coats of dusty rose polish and let dry for two minutes.

2. Wipe most of the dark burgundy polish off its brush, then paint small rectangular shapes in a tile pattern. Begin at the tip of the nail and vary the placement toward the base. Let dry for two minutes, then seal the design with top coat.

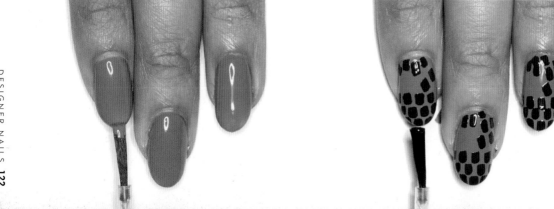

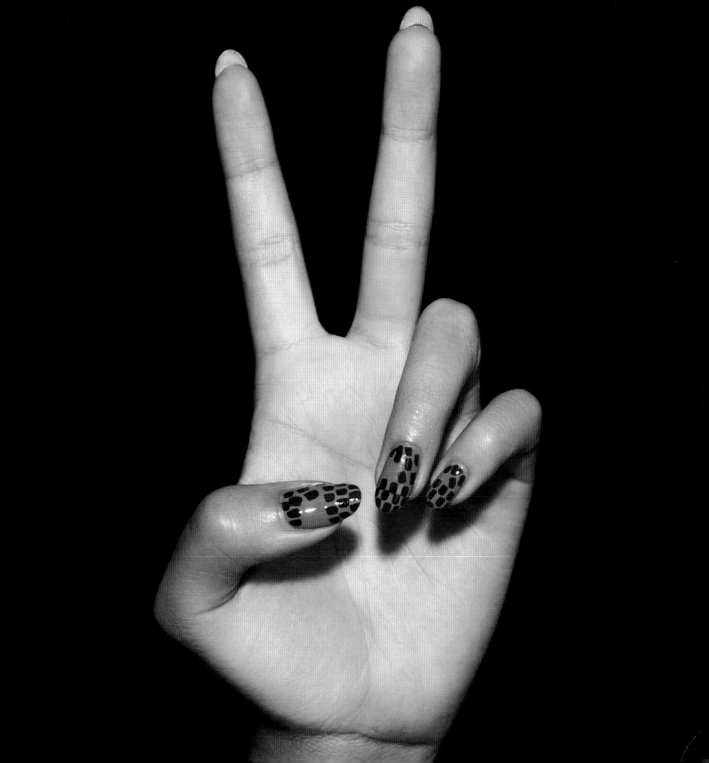

SOUND WAVES

This design features a single wave band across the nail, but you could also fill the entire nail with the design or vary the number of lines from nail to nail.

Tools

⌐ **Base coat**

⌐ **Bright peach polish**

⌐ **Fine art brush**

⌐ **Opaque black polish or acrylic paint**

⌐ **Top coat**

2. With a fine art brush and opaque black polish, paint squiggly lines across the nail horizontally. The line closest to the base of the nail should be a bit thicker than the rest. Let dry for two minutes, then seal the design with top coat.

1. Apply two coats of bright peach polish and let dry for two minutes.

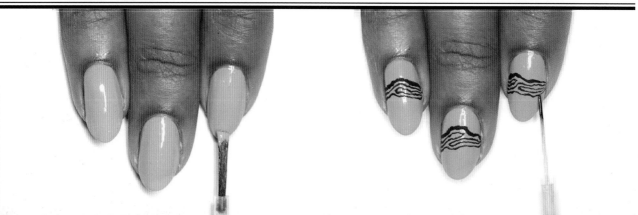

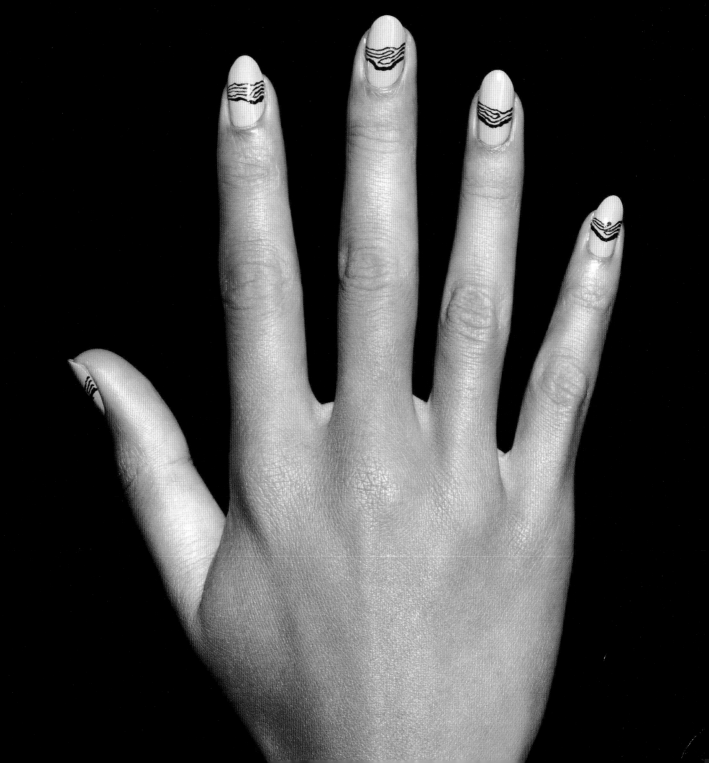

SPRAY PAINT

One of my most popular designs, this was inspired by the work of the great fashion designer Alexander McQueen.

Tools

¬ **Base coat**

¬ **Metallic gold polish with fine glitter**

¬ **Sheer black polish**

¬ **Thin fine art brush**

¬ **Opaque black polish or acrylic paint**

¬ **Top coat**

1. Randomly dab metallic gold polish with fine glitter all across the nail, leaving some open space in between. Let dry for two minutes.

2. Dab sheer black polish on some of the open spaces between the gold. Let dry for one minute.

3. With a thin fine art brush and opaque black polish, create a smaller blotch inside the sheer black dabs. Paint thin lines "dripping" toward the tip of the nail and add a few very small dots across the entire nail for greater effect. Let dry for two minutes, then seal the design with top coat.

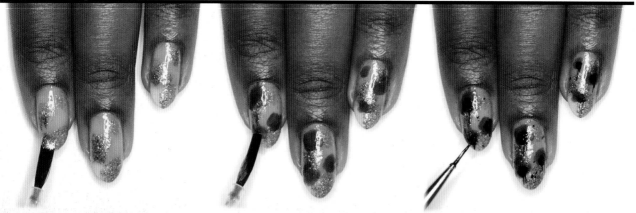

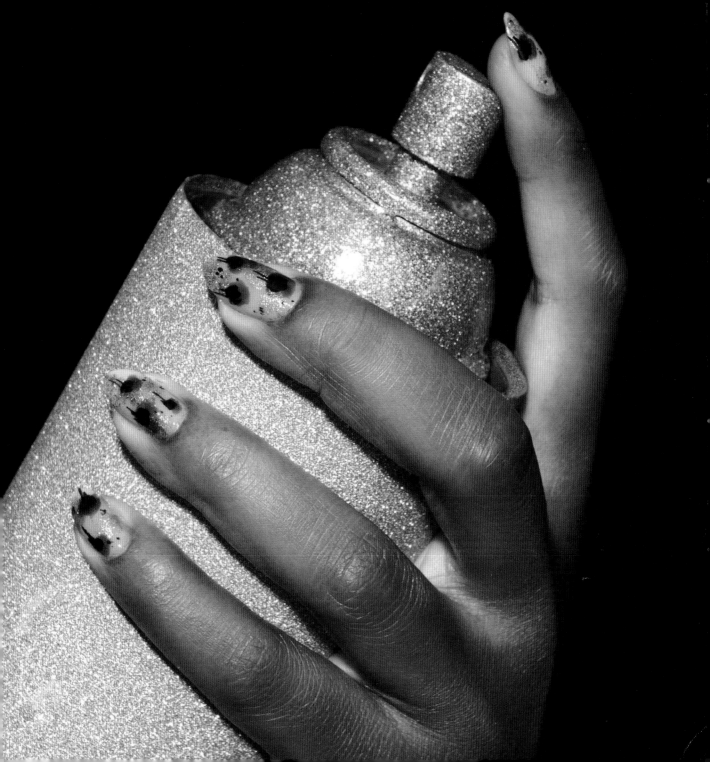

POP DOTS

I love the work of artist Keith Haring and tried to capture his Pop art style and the sense of movement in his work with this design.

Tools

- ☐ **Base coat**
- ☐ **Neon orange polish**
- ☐ **Opaque white polish or acrylic paint**
- ☐ **Thin fine art brush**
- ☐ **Opaque black polish or acrylic paint**
- ☐ **Top coat**

1. Apply two coats of neon orange polish and let dry for two minutes.

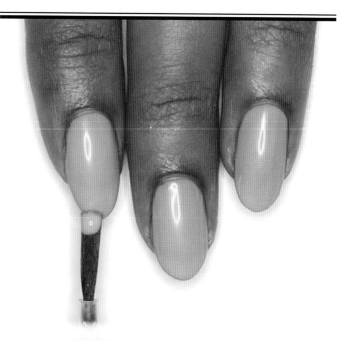

2. Working at an angle, paint random large spots of opaque white polish across the top half of the nail. Let dry for two minutes.

3. With a thin fine art brush, paint a small dot of opaque black polish inside each white dot and then outline the white dots with black as well. Let dry for two minutes.

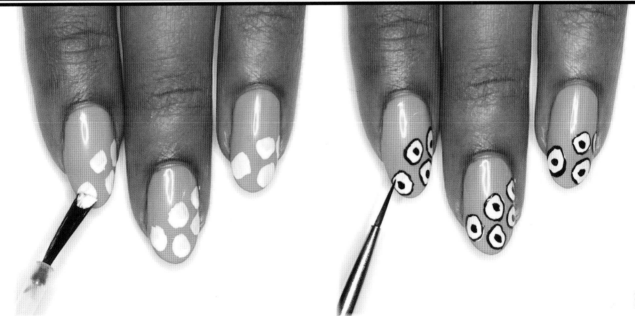

4. Keeping the same angle, use a thin fine art brush to paint tiny dots of opaque black polish between the larger dots. Let dry for two minutes, then seal the design with top coat.

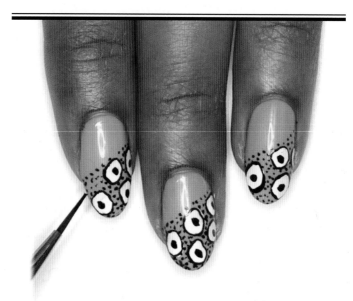

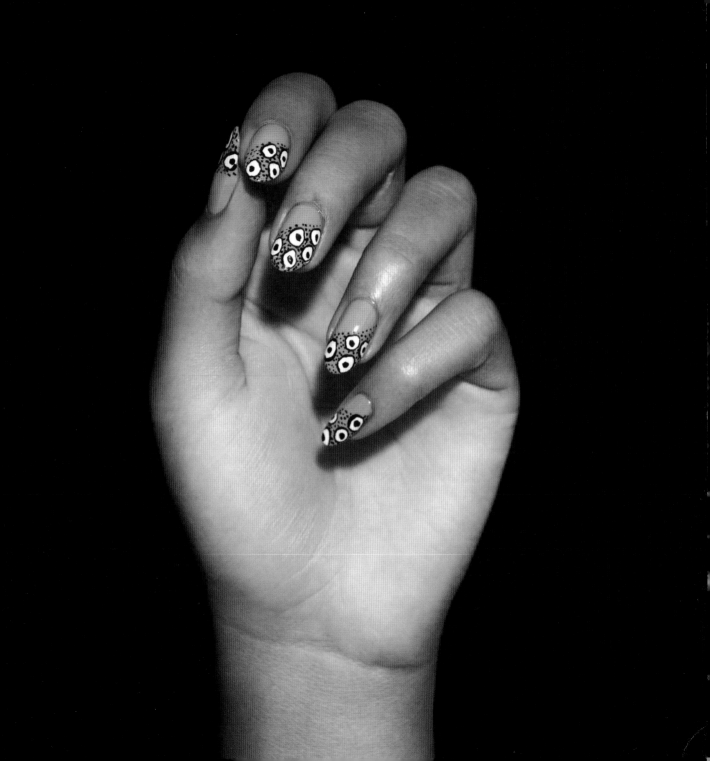

RESOURCES

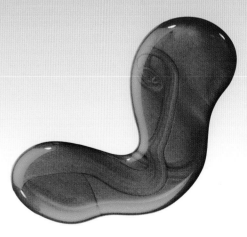

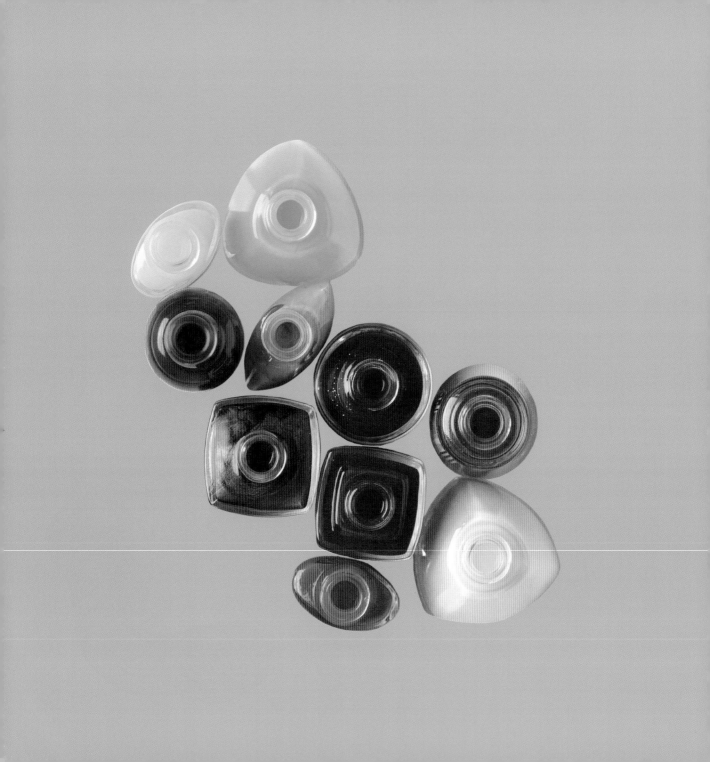

For more nail art inspiration, visit my blog at elsalonsito.com, or follow me on Instagram: @Amivnails. Some of my favorite polishes, which I used for this book and work with every day, are Zoya, DIOSA Nails & Polish, RGB, Essie, and Revlon—all available online. My favorite websites for nail art supplies are premiernailsource.com and fumicjewelrynail.com.

ACKNOWLEDGMENTS

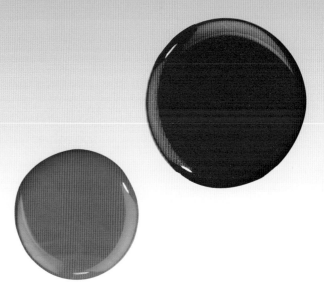

First I must thank the person who truly made this book happen, the person who worked day and night to make it come to life: my business partner and brother, Gabriel Vega. Thank you for making me believe in my talent and skills and for always being an encouraging voice when I needed it most. El Salonsito wouldn't be here without you. Love you!

Thank you to our parents, who support us in our pursuit for happiness in what we do; Gabriel and I are truly grateful for you. To those in my family who helped this single mama work the job that she loves by watching the little one, I am forever indebted to you. Thank you all for your continued support.

To the amazing crew who brought this book together visually, *thank you*! Jason Setiawan: thank you for capturing my work in ways unimaginable, and thank you for being such an amazing soul! The beautiful models Jessica,

Niove, Yinell, Ashley, and Linette: thank you for lending us your gorgeous hands and faces and for being such amazing canvases for my work. Mimi Wilson, you are amazing beyond words: thank you for being my second set of hands and for bringing the nail art into fruition. Candy Javier and Keisha Dale: you ladies truly worked your magic in this book with the makeup. I am forever indebted to each and every one of you.

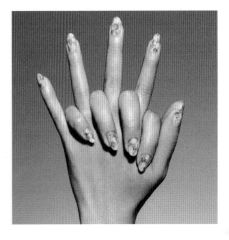

Gabe and I want to thank our literary agent, Stephany Evans—Stephany, thank you for all you've done and for your belief in our idea for this book. To our amazing writer, Marisa Bulzone: thank you so much for translating my ideas and words and for composing them into the beautiful book we have today.

To our editor, Jeanette Shaw; cover designer, Kaitlin Kall; and everyone at Perigee: thank you for bringing my dream to such beautiful fruition.